Prostate Cancer Came A Knockin'

A story of discovery, despair, determination, and divine intervention

Eric Otis Simmons

Disclaimer

Results from cancer treatment will vary, and no provider can guarantee a particular outcome. By purchasing this book, you acknowledge such. You will also hold harmless Eric Otis Simmons (Author of this Book, and hereafter referred to as Author) and the healthcare provider(s) mentioned in this title from any claims, lawsuits, demands, causes of action, liability, loss, damage and/or of every kind whatsoever, should you or anyone you share this book with receive a prostate cancer outcome or level of healthcare service dissimilar to that of the Author.

Aliases have been used to protect the privacy of the healthcare staff who cared for the Author. Therefore, any similarities in names are coincidental. Also, the conversations and medical information provided are from the Author's recollection and perspective and may differ.

The Purchaser hereby waives any and all claims arising from any actions or other activities or lack thereof by the Purchaser or any third party that may or may not have resulted from the content contained within this Publication. Furthermore, the purchaser agrees to indemnify and defend the Author, the Author's representatives, heirs, assigns, or designees against any and all claims by the Purchaser or any third party.

ISBN 9798985904765

Dedication

This book is dedicated to the men, their families, and loved ones impacted by prostate cancer. Our hearts and prayers are with you.

Acknowledgments

Thank you to my immediate family whose nicknames I've used in this book, my wife, Bay, and children, Dee, Pooh, and K.J. Your support before, during, and after my prostate cancer diagnosis has meant the world to me. I never knew how much you loved me and I of you until I was diagnosed with prostate cancer. You've given me the will to live and the courage to meet my disease head-on. And for that, and much more, I'm proud to call you my family!

I sincerely thank the Emory Healthcare and Winship Cancer Institute of Emory University staff for their care before and after my diagnosis. I'm acutely aware of some of the challenges COVID-19 presented you, yet, the masks you were required to wear couldn't hide the dedication and determination in your eyes to provide me with the best healthcare possible.

I also thank Dr. Linda Farries Cunningham for helping me navigate what I refer to as "These treacherous waters of prostate cancer." You being a sounding board and availing your experience as a pathologist to me has been invaluable during this challenging time.

Acknowledgments

Thanks also to Llawanna Faye Carroll for reviewing "Prostate Cancer Came A Knockin'" and providing valuable suggestions for improving the book.

And lastly, thank you to family members and friends for your thoughts and prayers, which I believe God is answering.

Table of Contents

Introduction

Imagine you're Daniel Eugene "Rudy" Ruettiger, the undersized walk-on football player at Notre Dame. Your grit, determination, and desire have enabled you to overcome immense obstacles, and your coaches, fans, and teammates admire you for these qualities. So heartwarming is your story; a movie is made with your nickname as its title. You're also a walk-on basketball player for the Fighting Irish, and during a practice, the team's best player twists his ankle and is out for the upcoming game against Alabama. So, after the workout, your Head Coach calls you into his office and says, "Rudy, you'll be starting tomorrow." After students learn the news, there's a buzz in the air, and a giant pep rally is held in front of "Touchdown Jesus," with shouts of "Rudy, Rudy" filling the air.

The next day, before tipoff, when the starting lineups are announced, you receive a rousing standing ovation when your name is called. Once the game begins, you're playing better than your Coach, teammates, or fans could have imagined. Then, suddenly during a timeout, the gymnasium lights go out. They continue to flicker off and on as they're being restored. Next, out of the dark, a shadowy figure eerily steps onto the court. You can't see the name on the back of the player's jersey, but this new "adversary" seems unimposing enough. Once the lights are restored and play resumes, however, you realize your foe is out of the ordinary and is adept at playing offense and defense. The rascal is as slippery as an eel and moves like an amoeba. First, he's over here; next, he's over there and plays dirty too! He just elbowed you in the groin on a scramble for a loose ball and never said a word.

Halftime comes, and Coach discusses the adjustments the team needs to make in the second half. Then, he tells each player whom they'll guard one by one. "Bill, you've got Scott Lewis. John, you've got Bob Henderson." After Coach tells your other two teammates whom they'll be defending, you say, "Coach, I guess that leaves me with the creepy guy that came off the bench. I couldn't read the name on the back of his jersey because it was smudged out. So, who's the player I'm guarding?" Coach replies, "Rudy, You've got Prostate Cancer!"

I use the example of Rudy as a basketball player intentionally as a lead-in to my story because, like my fictional counterpart, I was an undersized (5'7" and 147 pounds) walk-on college basketball player for a large University (Auburn). And, like Rudy, my grit and determination had endeared me to coaches, fans, and teammates. Another similarity is that we've heard the four dreaded words, "You've Got Prostate

Introduction

Cancer!" But unlike Rudy in my fictional account, my Prostate Cancer story is nonfiction, and my dilemma is real!

As background, I was one of those men who shied away from rectal exams because I felt they "violated" my manhood and had a homosexual connotation. And naively, as a former athlete, I thought my body was invincible and immune to a disease like cancer. Also, I arrogantly thought cancer happened to others and would never happen to me. So, when I turned fifty-five, my viewpoint was, "Why should I see a doctor to check my prostate if it requires a rectal exam? Why even bother with a checkup?" I also rationalized away that my dad had lived to ninety, and I didn't know of a single family member who'd ever had cancer. So I'd say to myself, "I'm good!"

Unfortunately, my machismo nearly cost me my life and still may. The consequences of my healthcare negligence and lack of regular prostate check-ups were severe to the extent that my wife and I both believe I would have died if I had waited much longer to see a doctor. Originally my tumor appeared confined to my pelvic region, but it has since spread to five areas of my body. Due to my "near death" experience with prostate cancer, I feel obligated to share my story with other men so that, prayerfully, they won't make the same mistake as me and will get regular prostate cancer checkups. Therefore, I'm hopeful "Prostate Cancer Came A Knockin"

Introduction

will serve as a "wakeup call" for men my age and that they'll get checked regularly for the disease because I wouldn't want anyone to go through or have to endure what I've experienced.

Chapter 1
You've Got Prostate Cancer

When I learned I had prostate cancer, it felt like I'd been instantly thrown into a bad dream and couldn't wake up. Immediately, I went into denial mode. Undoubtedly, there had to be something wrong with the hospital's scanner, or my medical records had gotten mixed up with someone else's. How could this be possible? As a former college athlete, I would imagine, like many of my peers who played at a high level, I thought my body was invincible. When injured, it healed quickly, had a high pain threshold, and hardly ever got sick! Plus, I was born with "good" longevity genes, and there was, to my knowledge, no history of cancer in my family. So yep, this was a mistake because cancer happens to other people, and there's no way it could ever happen to me!

Boy, was I wrong! After my prostate cancer was confirmed, I had loads of questions and tried rationalizing away how I could have ever gotten cancer in the first place. Some of my thoughts were:

'How could this happen? Was there something in the food I ate growing up?'

'Could drinking water from garden hoses when playing football as a youth have caused it?'

'Was the water I drank growing up part of the Tuskegee experiment?'

'Or was it brought on by the three decades of stress I was under as the only minority in most jobs I held with Fortune 500 companies?'

'Was it that keg party in college? You know, the one where I drank off the tap after a bunch of other dudes. Yeah, I got it from one of them.'

'Maybe one of my ancestors had cancer, and I inherited the gene.'

'I'm being punished for some sin(s) I committed.'

I nearly wore myself out racking my brain for answers, but there were no definitive ones. One of the things I'm convinced of is that some cells in my body have gone rogue, and they are wreaking havoc on me internally. The odd thing about this is that I don't feel sick, yet cancer is slowly eating away at my insides. And while I believe things happen for a reason and that we all have a purpose in life, I keep asking myself, 'What is the reasoning and intent behind my developing prostate cancer? Is God using me for a greater purpose, and if so, what is it?'

Since I don't know the answer to any of my questions, and probably never will, oddly, since my first hospitalization until now, something in my head keeps telling me to mentally capture everything happening to me related to my battle with prostate cancer and write it down. And with my medical records being accessible online 24/7, I can draw upon them to fill in any missing gaps. Perhaps, this mental prodding was intended for me to write this book because I'm a prime example of what could happen to men fifty-five and over if they fail to get checked annually for prostate cancer.

As I think about it, many men are probably like me in that they avoid having a rectal exam because, **in their mind, the procedure diminishes their "manhood" and has a perceived homosexual connotation**. Sadly, for some men, myself included, it might be both, and as a result, we tend to avoid seeing a doctor, especially when we know or suspect a finger might be inserted up our anus. This avoidance, I feel, is especially true for us Black men, who are 50% more likely to develop prostate cancer in our lifetime and twice as likely to die from the disease, per Memorial Sloan Kettering Cancer Center (MSK). Hopefully, my battle with prostate cancer will scare the hell out of men, even those in their forties, regardless of race, and incentivize them to get checked annually for prostate cancer. If caught early enough, prostate cancer is treatable, so why go through what I'm experiencing? So if you know a man that is hesitant about prostate cancer screening, I hope you'll share "Prostate Cancer Came A

Knockin'" with them. If my battle with prostate cancer saves one life, mentally capturing and writing down what I've gone through will have been worthwhile.

So how did I get to this point in the first place?

Chapter 2
A Not-So-Charmed Life

Since I was young, there have been times when it has felt like I've lived a "Charmed Life" because so many of my dreams have come true. I married the woman of my dreams, Bay, and our kids, Dee, Pooh, and K.J., have made us proud. And our grandchildren continue to make us even prouder. I excelled when others doubted me, traveled the world, and went from growing up with modest means to earning far more than my parents did.

I grew up being raised in a single-parent household by my Black mother. A brilliant woman with hours towards a Ph.D., I believe she purposefully "groomed" me so I would be adequately prepared to cope with life as a Black man in a predominately White America. My mother introduced me to the world beyond our home from an early age through my teenage years. She exposed me to things such as the arts, music, sports, and domestic air travel. The amount of "exposure" she provided me, I feel, was designed to help cultivate my worldliness and broaden my horizons as a thinker. Growing up, my Mom would play a dictionary word game with me to help me learn how to enunciate words correctly. She taught me which fork to use for my salad when dining at a formal dinner, how to pull a chair out and open a door for a lady, memorization skills, courtesy, and much more.

So I don't believe it surprised my Mom when I finished in the "Top 10%" academically of my high school and college graduating classes. Or when I walked on and made the basketball team at Auburn University. Or when I became the "first" Black hired in many of my various sales/sales management roles during my career tenure with some of America's "Most Admired" companies (IBM, AT&T, General Electric (GE), etc.). Or that I became the first Black class President of IBM's prestigious sales training program. Or that I opened previously closed doors to minorities at these companies.

By living up to one of my mother's principles, treating others as you would want to be treated, I achieved success as a minority during my career in Corporate America, despite facing insurmountable odds on numerous occasions. My domestic business travels took me to thirty-seven of our fifty states, and these visits helped further open my eyes to the viewpoints of others. Likewise, I learned how "open for business" other areas worldwide were during my international business travels. So my mom didn't seem surprised when I told her I had closed sales of $500,000 in Paris, $1,000,000 in Brussels, and $25,000,000 in Hong Kong because she'd "groomed" me to excel. These three sales, in particular, showed me that people in other countries didn't seem to care as much about my skin color as they do here in America. Instead, what mattered most, it seemed, were the skillset, business acumen, and competency I brought to the business table. Because I demonstrated these qualities consistently, I earned my customers' business, respect, and trust. And along the way, I gained a far greater appreciation for the opinion of others. So, until the day she died, my mother would beam with pride and tell me often how proud she was of me. Yes, I was living a "Charmed Life," indeed.

Throughout my life, I've also had two other resources to help guide me - one good, the other not. They are the two angels on my shoulders whom I first met when I was about four. They're tiny, like elves, and have wings. When I was young, they used to tap me lightly on my shoulders, but now they only speak to my mind. The one on the left is devilish, and the one on the right is angelic. Curious about the angel phenomenon I'd been experiencing since my youth, I researched Google for this book and learned, per Wikipedia, "In Islamic tradition, the two kiraman katibin are two angels called Raqib and Atid, believed by Muslims to record a person's actions… One angel figuratively sits on the right shoulder and records all good deeds, while the other sits on the left shoulder and records all bad deeds." And to think, when I told my Methodist mom about the angels on my shoulders, she probably brushed it off as mere childhood fantasies.

So with all of the blessings bestowed upon me, I was woefully unprepared when I got the news that I had cancer. I doubt anyone ever is. In an instant, I went from living a "Charmed Life" to a "Not-So-Charmed" one. My cancer diagnosis has left me feeling like I've been placed on death row and handed my death sentence, but I haven't been told the date yet. All I can do is pray and hope for a stay of execution. And as each day passes, all I can hear is the tick-tock of the clock of my life slowly winding down. I've gone from asking myself, 'How long will I live?' to 'When will I die?' Right now, death is looking me in the eye, and I can smell its breath! Well, so much for a "Charmed Life!" And where did my "caretaker" right shoulder angel go? Why is my world suddenly crashing down on me?

Chapter 3
My Yeast Infection

In 2017, four years before my prostate cancer diagnosis, I had a burning sensation for about a week whenever I urinated, and the pain was intensifying. Bay, whom I met my junior year in college, insisted I go to the outpatient clinic about a mile away, but I was convinced it was just a urinary tract infection and would subside soon. So, the next day, after updating my Memoir, "Not Far From The Tree," on my laptop in my basement office, I took a break and headed to the bathroom. As I started peeing, the pain was so intense that I screamed. After that, Bay rushed down the steps yelling, "Eric, are you okay?" She'd heard me from our second-floor bedroom! When she got to the basement door, moaning, I told her I was okay and still had difficulty urinating. Next, she said, "I don't know why you're being so hard-headed about going to the outpatient clinic." I replied, "Don't worry; I'm most definitely going after this experience."

What Bay didn't know was – that I was in so much pain and exhausted from peeing; I was sitting on the floor hugging the toilet bowl. Up until then, I never knew porcelain was so cold! As I was resting on the floor, I was trying to figure out what could have caused me to have a urinary tract infection that burns so badly! Wildly, I concluded it must have been the alcohol in beer since alcohol burns. Well, I never said I was a doctor. So, as I was blaming Bud Light for my dilemma, I started praying. 'Dear Lord, I promise you I'll never drink again if you relieve me of this pain. Amen.' After struggling to stand up, I washed my hands and grabbed my keys, wallet, and glasses before heading to the outpatient clinic. Once there, a nurse took me into an exam room and asked, "What brings you here today, Mr. Simmons?" "I think I have a urinary tract infection," I replied. "Okay, let me check your vitals first," she said. "After I finish, I'll need a urine sample, so before we get started, let me go and get a cup, and I'll be right back."

The nurse came back, checked my vitals, and, when she was done, handed me a cup to urinate in after she left. On her way out, she said, "Mr. Simmons, please stick your head out the door to let me know you're finished." After I said, "Okay," I closed the door behind the nurse, and when I tried to pee, a tear rolled down my right eye. First, a little bit of urine came out, then slowly, a little more. As it did, my urethra was on fire, and I could only pee enough urine to cover the cup's bottom. My urine was yellow and cloudy with some small white stringy things, which I figured were from my dead white blood cells fighting bacteria. When I was done, I called the nurse to tell her I was finished. When she returned to the exam room, embarrassed by my low urine output, I asked her, "Will this be enough?" She said it would.

About ten minutes later, the nurse returned and said, "Mr. Simmons, you are correct. Your white blood cell count is very high, and you have a urinary tract infection." Then out of nowhere, she asked, "Mr. Simmons, have you been having sex with someone other than your wife?" My first thought was, "What the f#*k!" Then, recognizing I was pissed off by the question and seeing an opening, my left shoulder angel quipped, "Say this. Why do you ask? Are you interested?" Exasperated, my right shoulder angel said, "Don't you dare say that!" So, I listened to my right shoulder angel and said, "No. I'm in so much pain; sex is the last thing on my mind."

Next, with a straight face, the nurse said, "Well, I thought it was worth asking. You've got all the symptoms of someone with an STD (sexually transmitted disease)." Now, I was about to blow a gasket! But instead, I inhaled, then exhaled and said, "I can assure you that's not the case." Then the angel on my left shoulder cleared his throat and whispered, "Go ahead. Ask her. I'm pretty sure she's interested." After that, my right shoulder angel flapped her wings wildly and said to the left shoulder angel, "Shut up, you moron! Now I see why you got kicked out of heaven."

While my angels were battling it out, the nurse continued her update.

"It turns out you have a yeast infection, Mr. Simmons."

"A yeast infection? Men don't get yeast infections!"

"I know it sounds strange, but it's true. About 2 to 3% of men get yeast infections."

"How the hell could I get a yeast infection? (The nurse gives me a look like, 'Well, you're the one with an STD, so you tell me.') So now I'm thinking, If this b*^#h answers, 'Well, maybe your wife is fooling around on you, I'll kick her ass'!"

Instead, she says, "Well, Mr. Simmons, various things, such as harsh soaps, an allergy, etc., can cause men to have yeast infections."

"Wow, I didn't know that."

"Most men don't."

After the nurse finished her update, I asked myself, 'Does this chick always have to have the last word?' So, when the nurse left to have the doctor write me an antibiotic prescription, I was still pissed that she thought I had an STD! But, by the time I got home, I'd cooled down. So, when I told Bay about the nurse's inquiry, we laughed. Then, as she was walking off, Bay nonchalantly said, "You should have asked her if she was interested." Next, and always the opportunist, my left shoulder angel kicked in and said, "See, I told you." Then, I started laughing so hard that I almost peed my pants.

A few days later, I was in Kroger getting some groceries, and I was so fascinated that a man could have a yeast infection I stopped a White lady who had just crossed in front of me with her buggy.

"Excuse me, ma'am. I don't mean to disturb you. I'm Eric, and you won't believe what happened to me the other day."

"Oh, Hi Eric, I'm Nancy. What happened?"

"Nancy, I found out I have a yeast infection!"

"Really?"

"Yes! About 2-3% of men get them."

"Well, now you men know what we women go through."

"I probably can't fully appreciate what women go through, but I did hug the toilet."

"Oh, that's nothing. I almost ripped ours out of the floor once!"

"Really?"

"Yes!"

"Wow!"

Next, Nancy spotted two other ladies and waved them over.

"Ladies, this is Eric, and he just shared with me that he has a yeast infection."

"Really?"

"Yes."

Soon, the three women and I were chirping about yeast infections like traders on Wall Street buying and selling stocks. During our back-and-forth exchange of yeast infection stories, Nancy spotted a fourth lady and waved her over. After that, the new arrival joined in on the chaotic conversation. And just like that, I'd become an unsung hero in these ladies' eyes for fessing up about my yeast infection, and I loved it!

After we all bid one another goodbye, I was proud to be an unofficial member of my local Kroger's Women's Yeast Club! Not long after I got home, Pooh dropped by, and I told her about my conversation with the ladies at Kroger. She said, "Lord Dad, I was telling my co-workers about you today. I said, "My dad is the only person I know who can go to Kroger, bump into the King of England, strike up a conversation, come home, and tell you all about what happened, and it would be true!" Then, Pooh and I had a good laugh.

Back then, my yeast infection story was funny. Today, however, it isn't because, several years after my yeast infection, I began getting out of bed five to seven times a night to urinate, started losing weight, and acquired a slight stomach bulge. While I didn't know what was causing my lack of appetite, I was convinced my new "pot belly" and frequent nightly urination were attributable to my getting older. In retrospect, my body may have been reacting to the initial stages of cancer and sending me a "warning" signal with the yeast infection.

Fast forward to Monday morning, November 22, 2021, and as I try to urinate, it's burning like hell. Quite naturally, I'm having a flashback to 2017. To make matters worse, I have a terrible case of indigestion. Again, and like with my yeast infection episode, Bay urges me to go to the outpatient clinic, but as I did then and had done for years, I ignored her advice about seeing a doctor. Noticing she's immensely frustrated and confused about my not wanting to see a doctor, I finally reveal to her my long-held secret.

"Bay, I never told you this, but when I was fourteen, my Mom asked my Dad to take me for a sports physical related to Junior High basketball tryouts. Unfortunately, the exam turned out to be a nightmare for me. As the male doctor was touching my genitals, I became increasingly uncomfortable. Being a teenage boy, having another male touch my private parts didn't seem right. Plus, it appeared to me that the doctor was enjoying it! So my hands began sweating profusely, and just when I thought I couldn't get any more anxious, the doctor asked me to bend over on an examination table so that he could give me a rectal exam. Now, I'm terrified."

"I couldn't see behind me, but I could hear his rubber glove snap as he put it on. Next, he told me he would apply a gel on his gloved finger before entering my anus. As the doctor's sizable finger entered my rectum, I squeezed my butt tightly to prevent his appendage's penetration. When he told me to relax, I tried but felt completely violated once his finger was inside me. I was so pissed off that I raised from the table and turned to punch him. As I was doing so, Dad ran over and caught my arm just before I could knock Doc's ass out! I scared the hell out of him and Dad. Startled, the doctor said, "This exam's over!" I thought to myself, 'You damn right it is!' Afterward, my emotions were all over the place. The genital touching and rectal exam constituted a homosexual act in my mind. I was so traumatized by the experience that I vowed that day that no man would ever touch my genitals or stick his finger up my butt again! Afterward, aside from sports physicals or similar that involved no genital touching or rectal exams, I stopped seeing a doctor."

After hearing my story, Bay pauses momentarily and says, "So that's why you don't like me touching your butt."

"Exactly!"

"But you athletes do it all the time."

"Yeah, but that's different.

"Why's it different?"

"It just is."

"But why?"

"Because they're my teammates, and a pat on the butt acknowledges a good play."

"Well, I'm your teammate too."

"Yes, you are, but you're a woman."

"What difference does that make?"

"A lot!"

"Why a lot?"

"It just does."

"Why? Where are you going?"

"Downstairs."

"Why are you going downstairs?"

"Because."

"Because what?"

"Because this conversation is giving me a headache, that's what."

When 1:00 P.M. rolls around, I'm in so much pain that I finally give in and say, "Bay, I'm going to the outpatient clinic." So, I head out, and after arriving at the clinic and checking in, a nurse takes me to an exam room a few minutes later. I tell her I'm having a burning sensation when I urinate, and I think I have a urinary tract infection. I also add that I'm experiencing severe indigestion. Next, the nurse asks for a urine sample and hands me a cup. After she leaves the room, I have to strain to pee. Nothing's coming out. After about five minutes of trying, a slight dribbling of urine finally drops into the cup. Exhausted, I open the exam room's door and call for the nurse to let her know I'm finished. When she comes back, I hand her the urine sample, and as I did in 2017, I figure I'll get some antibiotics plus something for my indigestion, and I'll be on my way.

After examining my urine sample, the nurse enters the exam room and says, "Mr. Simmons, you are right. Your white blood cell count is high, and you have a urinary tract infection. But there's something else. The doctor wants you to go to the emergency room right now!" I'm thinking, 'What the f*&k?' But, I say, "The emergency room? Why? What for?" The nurse replies, "Your bladder is so tight that we don't know what the problem might be. Unfortunately, we don't have a CAT scanner to help us determine the issue. So, the doctor wants you to go to the emergency room immediately!"

Dumbfounded, I tell the nurse, "I'll head to the emergency room right now," but when I leave the clinic, I head straight home. When I get home, after updating Bay about my clinic visit and the doctor's request, she's unhappy that I didn't go directly to an emergency room, so I tell her, "I'll go once rush hour traffic dies down." Truthfully, I'm stalling for time because I don't want to deal with any fricking doctors. Plus, I don't think anything is seriously wrong with me. So, like an idiot, I walk downstairs to my home office and pull up ESPN on my laptop. After an hour, I get up from my desk, go upstairs and tell Bay, "I'm heading to the emergency room, and I'll be back in a few hours."

Chapter 4
My Hospitalization

The double glass doors of the emergency room (ER) at my local Emory Healthcare facility open, and I walk in. The lobby is jam-packed, and everyone, except one or two, is wearing a mask because of COVID. After a short wait in line, I tell the receptionist, "The doctor at the outpatient clinic up the street told me to get to the emergency room immediately to have a CT scan done to see why my bladder is so hard." Next, the receptionist asks for my insurance card to make a copy, then hands me a clipboard with questionnaires and a consent form and tells me to bring them back to her when I finish. After completing the paperwork, I return the documents and clipboard to the receptionist. Then, she says, "You can be seated in the waiting area."

While sitting in the waiting room, my eyes and those of a woman across from me meet. So, I nod, say, "Hi," and start conversing with her. "I can't believe these many people are here on a Monday!"

"Me neither; this is incredible. I can't believe how long it's taking!"

"Yeah, COVID's got everything backed up. I've been here an hour and a half already."

"I came in after you, and I've been here an hour."

Next, I turn to my right, look at the teenager sitting next to me, and, shaking my head, repeat, "I can't believe how many people are here."

"Oh, it's always like this on Mondays. Mondays are one of the busiest days for an ER."

"How do you know so much about Emergency Rooms?"

"Sometimes, I have to go to an ER when my asthma medication runs out. Unfortunately, it's run out, and I'm not feeling well."

"Do you need me to get a nurse for you?"

"No, I'll be all right. Hopefully, I won't have to wait much longer."

"Let me know if you start feeling worse, and I'll get you a nurse."

"Okay, I will."

"Are you home for the holidays?"

"Yes, sir."

"You look like an athlete. Where do you go to school?"

"The University of Alabama. I'm a freshman, and I'm on their swim team."

"You've got to be kidding me. I apologize for laughing; I played basketball for Auburn."

"Really? That's too funny. I love going to the University of Alabama. I think it's the prettiest college campus in America."

There's no way I'm about to burst this ill young lady's bubble and tell her Auburn's campus is much prettier, so I say, "Yeah, you're right. Bama's campus is lovely. So, how are you managing your time between sports and school at Bama?"

"I'm adjusting pretty well. I have some friends from high school that go there, which helps some, but I don't see them much because I spend a lot of time with my swim teammates."

"That's great that you're adjusting so well! Most people have no idea how challenging it is to be a college student-athlete. We have to juggle sports, which is like a full-time job, and academics. It's a lot!"

"I agree. It is very challenging, and you don't have much time for a social life, so I love it when I come home and see my high school friends. Of course, I have friends at Alabama too, but I'm just starting to get to know them."

"While we've been talking, I've been thinking, so I have something to tell you."

"Really? What is it?"

"You're my hero."

"Really? No way! Am I? Why?"

"Well, you're a student-athlete competing at a high level for a Division I program in the grueling sport of swimming, which requires tremendous stamina, and, to top it off, you have asthma! That's incredible! Few people can do what you're doing, so you're my hero."

"Wow! Thank you so much!"

Next, the young athlete leans over, hugs me, rests her head on my chest, and starts crying. I pat her on her back and say, "There, there, now. I didn't mean to get you upset." "You didn't, she says. I'm just so happy right now." Then, with the young athlete crying in my chest, my eyes start welling up. I'm about to come unglued, and the lady across from me is about to lose it too.

So, when the young athlete's head finally lifts from my chest, I say, "You know what?" She replies, "No, what?" "You're not waiting a minute longer. I'm getting a nurse for you right now," I tell her. "Oh, no, please don't. I'll be okay," she says. "No, I insist," I assert. So, as I head to the reception desk, the student-athlete reaches to grab my arm but misses. I smile as I look back at her and say, "You missed. Too late!"

When I get to the reception desk, I raise my right arm to get the attention of one of the receptionists. I say, "Excuse me. I don't mean to be an alarmist, and I know the emergency room is jam-packed right now, but I think we may have a problem with that young lady over there, as I point to the student-athlete. Well, she's come to the emergency room because her asthma medication has run out, and over the last few minutes, I've noticed she's turned pale. So, I believe a doctor or a nurse needs to see her immediately." Then the receptionist looks across the lobby at the young woman and says, "Oh, my. Let me get someone out here right away. Thank you for letting me know."

When I return to my seat, I tell my fellow athlete, "Someone should be with you shortly." A few minutes later, a nurse appears from a light brown door to our right and calls the young girl's name. She says, "Here I am!" When she tries to stand, she's a little shaky, so I help her. I trail the nurse and student-athlete to the door where the nurse had come out, and before the nurse pushes a button to open it, the young athlete turns around, looks at me, and weakly says,

"Thank you." "Don't thank me," I tell her. "Get well because you're my hero." She smiles and walks through the door with the nurse; then it closes slowly behind them.

When I return to my seat, I look at the clock on my cell phone and discover I've been in the waiting area for two hours! Finally, a nurse enters the lobby and says, Eric Simmons. I stand and say, "Here!" The nurse escorts me through the same door the nurse and student-athlete went through, which leads to the ER. We turn left into a small room where the nurse checks my vitals. While doing so, she asks, "What brings you to the emergency room today, Mr. Simmons?" "I went to the outpatient clinic up the street for what I thought was a urinary tract infection, and they told me to get to an emergency room immediately to have a CAT scan done on my bladder, which they said was as tight as a drum. Since they didn't have a CT at their facility, they told me to come here immediately," I tell her.

After checking my vitals, the nurse leads me to a triage area with a curtain and a gurney. Once there, she tells me to remove all my clothes except my underwear. Next, she hands me a hospital gown to put on, and thirty minutes later, I'm rolled out on the gurney, taken into a room for a CAT scan, and then back to the triage area. I'm sitting on the gurney when an emergency room doctor pulls back the curtain, closes it, introduces herself, and says, "Mr. Simmons, as an update, you've suffered acute renal failure! If you had waited much longer, you probably would have had to have been placed on dialysis. So we will immediately admit you into the Intensive Care Unit for further tests and evaluation." I'm in total disbelief about the news, and as I look at the doctor, I'm thinking, 'B*^#h; you're lying! There's no f*#kin way my kidneys have failed. I feel fine!' I'm convinced the scowl on my forehead and glare in my eyes startles her because Doc quickly pulls open the curtain and hurries out of my small triage "room." I'd later learn my kidneys were functioning at only a 6% Glomerular Filtration Rate (GFR), considered Stage 5 Chronic Kidney Disease (CKD). I also learned patients with a GFR score of 15 or less are considered candidates to start dialysis therapy or be considered for a kidney transplant, per the National Kidney Foundation. So I was in a precarious position in the ER right off the bat!

A few minutes later, the nurse who took my vitals walks into my "room." Seeing I'm immensely disturbed by the doctor's update, the nurse does her best to calm me down. "My apologies, Mr. Simmons," she says. "Sometimes, doctors don't quite know what to say or how to convey what may be disturbing news to patients. You're going to be just fine." After the nurse leaves, I feel a little better and think my situation might not be as dire as the doctor has made it out to be. At least, I hope that's the case.

As I'm trying to digest the news I've received about my bladder and kidneys these past four or five hours, I scoot back on the gurney to try and sort things out. I'm wondering what could be going on with my body. Bewildered, I'm shaking my head side to side in disbelief when suddenly, out of nowhere, a bright light about three feet in circumference and coming from the ceiling appears in the curved right corner of the overhead u-shaped curtain track going around my "room." Thinking a fluorescent light has short-circuited, I look up and around at the fluorescent lights in the ER for as far as I can see, and none within my line of sight are nearly as bright as the one in my "room." I'm beginning to realize something is happening that isn't "normal." As I look at the light, there's a divineness to it. It's as if heaven has opened up and put a spotlight in the corner of my "room." Aware I'm fully coherent, I mumble, 'I'm completely lucid right now,' to myself. 'You've got to concentrate on everything happening right now and mentally capture it because no one will believe you when you tell them what you're experiencing.'

I sense a presence among the bright light, but I can't see it. The "aura" feels like it's emanating around the outer perimeter of the beam. I'm confused because, in the movies, a bright light comes toward you when you're about to die, but this one is pointing downward. As I look at the beam, it feels like I'm being watched and assessed by it. I can't see God's face, but I'm sure it's Him, and it's as though He's looking in on me right now. I'm not saying a word or moving because I don't want to startle the light and cause it to disappear. So I wonder, 'Why is the light only appearing in my "room" and no other place in the ER?' These past few hours have been so mentally draining; my head drops from my tiredness. With tears rolling down my cheeks, I shake my head in disbelief, and as I resign myself to my fate, I say, 'Oh no, Lord. I can't believe I'm about to die. I feel just fine. My kidneys don't even hurt. It just doesn't seem like it's my time yet. If it is your will for me to die, may your will be done.' Instantly, I'm no longer afraid to die. God has come to get me, so there's no need to fight it. Next, when I lift my head to look at the light again, time stands still as I wait for what will happen next. Also, I can't hear a sound in the emergency room. After a short while, the light slowly fades away, and when it does, I think, 'God just looked into my room and said, Oh, that's Butch (my nickname); I'm not ready for him yet.' Relieved that it isn't my time to die, I realize I've just experienced an epiphany or "divine moment" and feel assured I'll be okay no matter what is wrong with me. Next, I'm suddenly overcome with sadness, however, because if it isn't me that's about to die, I'm sure someone close to me in the emergency room will pass away tonight. But I don't know who it will be. I can't see the person to my left because the curtain is drawn, but I see a Black man in the "room"

next to me on my right. I hope it's not him

Following my "bright light" experience, the emergency

room doctor returns and says, "Mr. Simmons, my apologies if

I startled you earlier. Let me give you a better idea of what's

going on. Your CAT scan revealed your bladder is extended

almost to your sternum. Your bladder has been retaining

urine for so long that it's backed up your kidneys, and right

now, they are functioning at only a six percent (6%)

level. Currently, all the rooms in the hospital are filled with

COVID patients, but because your situation requires

immediate attention, we're designating this space as an

"intensive care room." I'll have a nurse put a catheter in you

so we can begin draining your kidneys immediately." Hearing

the news about the catheter insertion, I ask, "Are you going

to use anesthesia to sedate me? I know I'll pass out if you

don't." The doctor replies, "No, you won't need anesthesia."

Next, a nurse walks in and starts getting ready to insert a

catheter in me. I tell her nicely, "Look, if you're going to put

anything up my penis (I want to say dick head), you'll have to

put me under because I know mentally I won't tolerate the

pain. There's no chance I'll be able to handle this without

being sedated." So, she says, "Don't worry, Mr. Simmons,

I've done these hundreds of times. It might hurt a little

initially, but trust me, you'll be okay." Then, when I see the wording fourteen (14) inches written on the catheter's packaging, I immediately think, 'The Hell you say! If you stick that damn thing up my penis, I'll pass out and shit myself!'

After preparing the catheter, the nurse says, "Now, take a deep breath." When I do, she begins inserting the catheter. It feels like a red-hot poker is going through the head of my penis and urethra. I'm starting to see white stars flashing before my eyes. When the catheter hits what I later learned is my sphincter muscle, I'm damn near ready to pass out. After the nurse gets the catheter into my bladder and pee starts flowing into a urine bag beside the bed, she says, "Now there. That wasn't so bad." If I weren't so exhausted from the catheter insertion and she were a man, I would knock his ass out! That hurt like hell! So, I tell the nurse, "If any of you ever need to stick another catheter up in me, you'll have to put me under, so I won't feel it." The nurse replies, "There, there now," which is of little comfort to me. When she leaves, my first thought is, 'The CIA doesn't need to water torture our enemies. Instead, they could stick a catheter in them, and the prisoners of war would tell it all. If I were one of the captives, and they inserted a catheter in me, I'd give away all the military positions. I'd even tell them the location of the attaché case with the codes to the nuclear button!'

Finally, it dawns on me that I've been at the hospital for about three hours and haven't updated Bay. So trying not to yell, I call out in the ER, "Nurse. Oh, Nurse." After one comes, I ask, "Would you please have someone call my wife so she knows I'm being admitted? I left her number at the desk when I checked in." The nurse says, "Will do, Mr. Simmons." About thirty-five minutes later, when Bay arrives at the hospital, I don't know who's more worried, her or me. She's brought me something from Chic-fil-A because I told her I was starving when we spoke over the phone. I quickly wolf down my chicken sandwich but don't eat my fries because they're cold. Bay's so visibly shaken up about me that I don't have the heart to tell her about the cold fries.

When I stand up to look for someplace to throw away my trash, my gown comes untied in the back. I'm struggling to retie it, so Bay says, "Here, let me help you. When she finishes, I say, "Bay, you won't believe what happened to me. I'm sure no one will. A bright light appeared in the corner of the "room" right over there. I'm sure it was God looking in on me." After Bay says, "I believe you, Eric," I tell her, "Whatever's wrong with me, because of the bright light, I know I'll be all right. I can't explain it, but I know I will." After that, as I sipped on the Sprite with the meal Bay had brought me, the ER doctor and nurse who catheterized me entered my "room." First, they introduce themselves to Bay.

Then after the introductions, the doctor says, "We'll take you upstairs for a cystoscopy to see what's going on with your bladder and perform a similar procedure for your kidneys. So now, I'll have the nurse give you a pill that will cause you to sleep." I say, "Okay," and after the nurse gives me the medication, I use my Sprite to help me swallow it. After that, the nurse unlocks the gurney's wheels, and as she's wheeling me out of the "room," Bay is beside me on my right and is about to cry. Just as the double doors open leading out of the ER, I can feel my eyes get heavy then everything goes black.

When I wake up, I'm in a bed in a hospital room. I'm a little woozy and have tubes hanging out of both arms. To better view my new surroundings, I raise my head off my pillow and use both hands to help me sit up. As I'm getting myself into a comfortable position, my penis is incredibly sore, so I pull back the white blanket covering me and lift my hospital gown to take a look. Blood is on the tip of my penis, and some has dripped onto a blue pad underneath me. When I bend over to look closer, I trigger the alarm on the IV machine on my left. The beeping is driving me crazy, so I start pressing buttons on the unit's front panel, but nothing happens. Finally, I locate and press the nurse call button on the remote control that raises and lowers the bed I'm on and turns the tv off and on. Soon, a nurse comes into the room and mercifully stops the IV machine from its incessant noise. She resets the device and adds some fluid to the IV bag, which has a long rubbery plastic tube that ends with a needle in the bend in my arm. I tell her that I remember being taken out on a gurney, and now that I'm awake, I'm in a hospital room with tubes in my arms and blood coming out of my penis. I ask, "What happened?" She tells me I had to have an emergency cystoscopy as if I know what the hell that is. Then, seeing I'm confused, she says, "Your urologist will explain it to you." I think, 'Huh! Urologist? What urologist?'

After the nurse leaves, one-by-one hospital staffers come into my room. First, a technician to draw my blood, then a doctor, then a kidney specialist, then another tech to check my vitals, and then a nurse. There's so much going on that my head is spinning. Finally, the last person at the end of the "parade" is a female urologist with a lovely African accent who begins conversing with me about my status.

"Hello, Mr. Simmons. I'm Dr. Aminu. How are you feeling?"

"Exhausted!"

"Well, you've been through a lot. Why don't I give you an update on things?"

"Sure."

"Well, you've got an obstruction that's not allowing you to urinate, and it's also impacted your kidneys. So you had to have an emergency cystoscopy. It's a procedure where we go up the urethra and inside the bladder using a thin camera to see what is going on internally. Also, to further help your kidneys, I tried, for two hours, to place ureteral stents to help urine pass from your kidneys to your bladder but was unsuccessful. Typically, the procedure takes forty-five minutes to an hour. So, for now, the catheter is in place to help you urinate and to help your kidneys start to improve". Then, when Dr. Aminu says, "In addition," my thought is, 'What there's more?' "I'm concerned about your creatinine and PSA (Prostate-Specific Antigen – a test used to screen for prostate cancer) levels being so high. And your prostate appears enlarged on your CT scan, so I'd like to give you a rectal exam."

I'm thinking, 'Wow! I've got a lot going on that's wrong with me. And to top it off, she wants to give me a rectal exam! Please, not one of those!' So, when I ask her, "When?" she says, "Now!" At this point, I'm so mentally, physically, and emotionally drained from the past twenty-four hours that I don't see how things can get any worse. Plus,

I'm at peace with whatever is wrong with me because I believe the bright light I saw was heavenly "assurance" that everything would be all right.

Before the rectal exam, I'm trying to think of a way to win Dr. Aminu over, so she'll be gentle with me during my examination. Hoping that she might be from Nigeria, my first thought is, since my DNA results from four years ago revealed I'm predominately Nigerian, I'll play my "Who knows, we might be cousins" card to establish a connection with her. So I begin a conversation.

"Where in Africa are you from, Dr. Aminu?"

"I'm from Nigeria."

"Really?" (Now it's time for me to play my 'We might be cousins' card). "Several years ago, I took a DNA test, which revealed I'm 38 percent Nigerian."

"That's nice."

After hearing Dr. Aminu's response, I'm thinking, 'What? Are you kidding me? That's nice. That's it? Just a that's nice?' And to think I was just about to drop my; 'Who knows, we might be cousins line,' and all she can say is, "That's nice." Well, I'm pretty sure my plan to try and win her over has just backfired. More concerning to me is - based on the look in her eyes, I think I just pissed her off. She's looking at me like, 'Yeah. So go ahead and drop your; Hey, we might be African cousins card if you want to. I'll feed your scrawny butt to one of the lions back home!'

'Is it not cool for an African American to acknowledge they're from Africa to a native African? Geez, I don't know. I hope I haven't offended her because if I have, she may take it out on my rectum and use more than one finger. Or worse, insert her whole fist up my butt during the rectal exam! Wait a minute. Maybe I'm overreacting here. Perhaps we're not hitting it off due to our cultural differences. Yeah, that's got to be it. 'Nah. That's not it. She's pissed. I don't think she likes me. I'm pretty sure of it. But what if I'm misreading her, and she's just the consummate professional? Yeah, that's it. Ever since she walked into the room, she's been all business and no-nonsense. She's concerned about my health and wants to keep things professional. That's got to be it.'

So after my faux pas, Dr. Aminu says, "Mr. Simmons, I'd like you to get into a fetal position." So I do. After lubricating her gloved finger with gel, she begins the rectal exam. After she moves her finger through my anus and starts pushing and moving my prostate around, it hurts some, but it's bearable. This examination isn't nearly as bad as what I recall from my teenage sports physical. Maybe it's because Dr. Aminu is a woman; I don't know. Right now, I'm so worn out from giving blood, having monitors beeping, and nurses waking me up to drain my catheter bag that I could

give a damn about having a finger up my ass. Dr. Aminu

must be a mind reader because just as I had finished my

thought, her finger went up so far in me that I yelled, "Ow!"

Next, she says, "Mr. Simmons, your prostate feels

enlarged." Well, now I'm thinking, 'You should know,

doc. Your finger's been so far up in me that it also said hello

to my tonsils.'

After Dr. Aminu finishes my rectal exam, she tells me

she'll have more blood work ordered to see if my PSA level is

improving. Then she hits me with something out of the

blue.

"You know, Mr. Simmons. I've been thinking about

how we might be able to help your kidneys. Since going

up through your urethra was unsuccessful, I think we

should try to work down to your kidneys to assist your

urination process further. So the procedure I'm thinking

about will involve placing nephrostomy tubes internally

and attaching them to both kidneys to aid in draining

your urine should your kidneys begin to fail. So I would

like for you to think about that. Any questions?"

With tears welling up in my eyes, I say, "No," but then I add,

"I'm just so tired right now. Everything is happening so fast. I can't believe all of this is going on. I'm a former college athlete. I'm not supposed to get sick. Something like this isn't supposed to happen to me. Up until a day or so ago, I felt fine. But now that I think about it, maybe my body sent me warning signs that I ignored. I need time to think about it; what did you say those tubes are called again?"

"Nephrostomy tubes."

"Yes, those."

After Dr. Aminu leaves, despite my being physically and emotionally drained when Bay returns to the hospital, I update her on my condition as best I can. As I wrap up, I add, "I don't think the urologist likes me." Perplexed, Bay says, "What makes you say that?" "Well, she's from Nigeria, so I tried to connect with her by sharing that I'm about thirty-eight percent Nigerian. There was no reaction. I don't know, but I think I may have offended her," I reply. Then, out of nowhere, Bay starts crying. "What's the matter?" I ask. "Please don't worry about me. I'm going to be all right," I inform her. Next, she slowly turns away from the window she's been staring out of and tells me Juanita, one of her youngest sisters, has just passed away. Shocked by the news, I reply, "What? Oh no, Bay, I'm so sorry to hear that!" Before I can say anything else, Bay turns back towards the window she's been looking out and uncontrollably starts crying while lifting her hands heavenward in prayer.

Seeing Bay cry causes my heart to sink, and suddenly I'm angry and resentful about my hospitalization. My wife needs me more than ever, and I'm stuck in a hospital bed! Why now and at a time like this? There's absolutely nothing I can do to help her. Lord knows I don't want my hospitalization to burden her further as she's mourning the loss of her sister. I've never felt so helpless in my life.

After Bay leaves, Pooh, a Doctor of Physical Therapy, and K.J., who recently graduated with a Master's in Speech-Language Pathology, arrive. Dee, a College Assistant Baseball Coach, lives out of state, so Bay and his siblings are keeping him updated on my situation. I tell Pooh and K.J. not to worry about me and that I'll be okay. I add, "The best thing you can do for me right now is to be there for your Mom. She was already struggling with my hospitalization, and now she's devastated over losing one of her sisters. So I need you guys to promise me you'll care for your Mom because I can't do it now." After hearing my request, the two tell me not to worry and say they'll care for their Mom in my absence. They also add they want me to concentrate on improving, and I tell them I will.

As Thanksgiving nears, my kidney function has improved somewhat from 6% to 9% GFR, and my creatinine level has declined from a high of 8.25 mg/dl to 5.18 mg/dl, which are somewhat encouraging signs. Still, I'm far from being out of the woods. As a result, the morning shift attending physician tells me I'll need to stay in the hospital through Thanksgiving, which is terrible news because this will be the first time I've ever been away from Bay and the kids on Thanksgiving.

About an hour later, the phone in my room rings, and when I answer, it's Dr. Aminu.

"Hello, Mr. Simmons. How are you feeling?"

"Much better, thank you."

"Mr. Simmons, I'm still worried about your creatinine level and kidneys. Have you had time to think about the nephrostomy tubes I mentioned?"

"No, not really, because we just got the news that one of my wife's sisters has passed away."

"I'm so sorry to hear that."

"Thank you. If you feel God is leading you toward the nephrostomy tubes, I'm okay with that." The phone goes silent for a few seconds, and then Dr. Aminu says,

"Let me think about it some more."

"Okay."

About two minutes after hanging up with Dr. Aminu, the phone in my room rings again. I'm pretty sure it's her calling back, so before I answer, I think, 'God sure answered Dr. Aminu's call quickly!' When I pick up the phone, it is her, and she begins by saying, "Mr. Simmons, the more I think about it, the more I think we should go with the nephrostomy tubes." So, without hesitating, I tell her, "If that's where you feel you're being led, let's do it." "Okay, I'll set it up," she says.

After hanging up, the first thing that comes to my mind is, 'Since the doctors were having difficulty pinpointing what was going on with me and my prostate appears to be enlarged, I must have prostate cancer. That's the only thing that makes sense. Surely they must expect I have cancer, and if so, why are they not looking to remove my prostate? The upside to this, I suppose, is that they aren't coming in here and wanting to cut on me to make a buck. But my dad didn't have cancer, and I don't know anyone in my family that has ever had it, so if I've got it, it has to be a "one-off."' With Bay worrying about me and dealing with her sister's death right now, I won't tell her and the kids that I think I might have prostate cancer. So, for now, I'll remain positive in their

presence and keep my suspicions about having cancer
to myself.

On Thanksgiving day, Bay, Pooh, and K.J. stop by the
hospital to see me. They tell me their day hasn't been the
same with me not being at home, but otherwise, they've had a
quiet and as enjoyable day as best they can muster. When
Dee calls, it's apparent he's shaken and worrying about me, so
I have to lift his spirits. When Bay, Pooh, and K.J. leave, I'm
saddened and start crying. After night falls, I can't go to sleep
because I'm constantly being wakened for bloodwork or to
have my urine bag emptied, so at about 11:00 P.M., I'm
clicking through channels on my room's tv, and the Weather
Channel pops up. It says there's light rain and fog in my area.
How ironic that the forecast mirrors my mood and spirit right
now. However, mine is much gloomier than the weather
prediction.

A few days pass, and Dr. Aminu drops by to see me to
update me on my status. She tells me the nephrostomy tubes
are scheduled to be placed on Monday, November 29th at
9:00 A.M. She reassures me the tiny tubular catheters are a
precautionary step and will only be used if my kidneys fail.
She also tells me she's confident that if my kidneys continue
progressing, the tubes won't have to be used - but reasserts
it's better to be safe than sorry.

Chapter 5
Nephrostomy Tubes Placement

On Monday, the 29th, two nurses come to my room to take me to Interventional Radiology (IR) for a doctor to place my nephrostomy tubes. First, they help me slide over from my bed onto a gurney; then, they wheel me out of my room and onto an elevator. When we get on the elevator, one of the nurses pushes the down button for us to head to the hospital's basement, where IR is located. Once there, I'm wheeled into a small room on the left, across from the nurses' station. After the two get me settled in the room, an IR nurse, working alone at the station, enters and introduces herself. She tells me a little about the nephrostomy procedure I'm about to have and says she'll be in the surgical room assisting Dr. Bellinger, who'll be placing the tubes. When the nurse finishes her overview, she asks me if I need anything, and shivering, I say, "A warm blanket would be nice. I'm freezing!" "I understand," she says. "By us being in the basement, it does get cold down here."

After a few minutes, the nurse returns with two heated blankets, in which I try to wrap myself up like a mummy to keep warm. "These feel great," I tell her, "And I'm not nearly as cold as before." Before heading out the door, the nurse tells me Dr. Bellinger should be with me shortly.

About fifteen minutes later, someone knocks on the door, and a woman wearing a hospital "white coat" enters and introduces herself. "Hello, Mr. Simmons, I'm Sandra Bellinger; it's nice to meet you," she says. "The pleasure's all mine," I state.

While Dr. Bellinger tells me what will happen during the procedure, I'm impressed with her intellect and bedside manner. Most doctors, it seems, possess the former but not the latter. Her words are comforting to me because before coming to IR, I was extremely apprehensive about having tubes placed inside me that may never be used. When she finishes telling me about the procedure, Dr. Bellinger asks if I have any questions, and after telling her, "I don't," I say, "I find your bedside manner and demeanor most impressive. I'm confident I'm in good hands with you." (Hey, if someone is about to cut on me, I should butter them up first!). "You've put my apprehension and anxiety at ease about having tubes placed inside me." "Thank you," she says. "I'm glad I have." Next, the assisting nurse knocks on the door and says, "Dr. Bellinger, can I see you for a minute?" Dr. Bellinger excuses herself and, when she returns, says, "I'm so sorry for having to step out, Mr. Simmons. Unfortunately, the emergency room is overflowing, and I just got called to perform an emergency procedure. So, I'm going to have the nurse take you to a room, and hopefully, I'll be back in about an hour or so."

After Dr. Bellinger leaves, the nurse rolls me and the gurney I'm on into a room to the right of the nurses' station, with a bed and tv. About an hour after I've settled in, I notice my urine bag is full. So I wriggle out of my bed and head down the hall to the restroom, holding my urine bag in my left hand and the back of my hospital gown in my right to keep the nurses and other patients from seeing my naked butt. Because it's quiet as a mouse in the IR, I grow increasingly embarrassed with each of my steps because you can hear the swish, swish, swishing sound of my urine moving around inside the bag. So, as I'm waddling down the hall like a duck to keep my urine bag quiet, I'm sure I'm a sight to see. I'm thinking, 'I can't wait to be rid of this catheter.' After I drain my urine bag, I head back to my room, relieved there's no more swishing sound as I walk, and get back onto my bed, where I fall asleep watching tv.

After waking up, I pick up my cellphone to look at the time and am stunned to see it's 1:00 P.M.! I've been waiting in IR for four hours! Upset, I press the call button, on the remote, for a nurse. Upon entering the room, the attending nurse says, "I'm so sorry, Mr. Simmons. We haven't forgotten about you. Unfortunately, we're so swamped with COVID patients; everything is backed up. Dr. Bellinger is still in surgery. I'll let you know as soon as I learn about her availability. In the meantime, can I get you anything?" "Well, I'm not too happy about this," I express. So, the nurse says, "I understand." Next, I tell her that since I'm still limited to graham crackers and liquids; I'd like a pack of graham crackers and a Sprite. "Sure," she says. "Since we've kept you waiting so long, I'll bring you two of each." "That's great," I say.

After the nurse leaves, I call Bay with an update and share, "I don't think they'll be able to get to me today, so you can come and pick me up. I know the hospital's busy with COVID patients, but this is ridiculous! I've been here for four hours!" Knowing I'm somewhat impatient and tend to have a short fuse, especially regarding tardiness, Bay says to me sternly, "Eric, calm down! Just calm down. You know you can't leave, so just be patient. I'm sure they'll get to you as soon as they can." After being put in my place by Bay, but still wanting to have the last word, I say, "Yeah, I guess you're right. But this is ridiculous!" Then Bay shouts, "Eric!" "Okay, okay," I sheepishly reply.

I fall asleep again and am awakened by a knock on my room's door. When I say, "Come in," in walks Dr. Bellinger, who says, "Oh, Mr. Simmons. I'm so sorry. The emergency room had several patients that required immediate surgeries, so I had to perform back-to-back operations. But I'm ready for you now." Groggy from just waking up, I ask, "What time is it?" "It's 4:00 P.M.," she says. "I'll get myself prepped and see you there." After Dr. Bellinger leaves, the attending nurse returns to wheel me into the procedure room. Once there, I sense a high degree of urgency from Dr. Bellinger and the nurse to complete the placement of my tubes because I think they feel terrible about the seven hours it has taken to get to me.

When we get to the procedure room, which must be a new name for a surgery room, a male anesthesiologist and another female nurse await. The two nurses help me slide off my gurney onto a surgical table. Next, they roll me over onto my stomach, and one has me place my chin in a stirrup. After that, the other uses a large Q-Tip to rub a liquid on my back "to numb it," she says. The fluid is so cold that the other nurse brings me a warm blanket when she notices I'm shivering. Next, the anesthesiologist asks me what type of music I like, and when I say "Rhythm and Blues," he says, "Coming right up!" I can't see where he goes when he leaves, but music starts playing in the room within less than a minute. After the anesthesiologist returns, I say, "Ahh, Frankie Beverly. Very nice!" Then, he tells me, "I'm about to put an oxygen mask over your nose and mouth, so I want you to breathe normally. After a few minutes, you're going to feel very relaxed. We aren't putting you to sleep, however.

You'll be awake during the procedure, so if you have any questions, feel free to ask us." Surprised I'd be awake during the surgery, I jokingly remark, "If I'm going to be awake during the process, that's got to be some good "happy juice" you've got going on there." After my comment, the anesthesiologist and nurses have a good laugh.

Next, Dr. Bellinger starts getting her "team" organized. She sounds like a drill sergeant as she sets her expectations of the others. It's as if she's saying, 'Listen up. I'm bringing my A-game, so I expect the same from each of you!' As I'm listening to Dr. Bellinger as she "barks" instructions, there's no doubt who's in charge in this room, and I can sense everyone has gotten the message too. I'm waiting for someone to say, "Aye, Aye, Captain."

As Dr. Bellinger begins the procedure, she and I are conversing. Step by step, she's telling me everything she's doing and, at one point, says, "I'm about to make two small incisions." When she does, I don't feel a thing. "Yep," I express to the anesthesiologist, "This "happy juice" works! I can't feel a thing." Next, I start getting giddy and very chatty. Now, I'm conversing with everyone in the room, and before I know it, Dr. Bellinger says, "I'm done!" When I ask her how long the procedure took, she says, "Oh, about forty-five minutes." I reply, "It seems like it has only been ten, no more than fifteen minutes." "Well, you did great," she says.

"The nurses will get you ready to go back to your room. It was a pleasure meeting you." "It was a pleasure meeting you as well," I tell her.

When the nurses turn me over onto my back, I feel two rigid pieces of plastic "tubes" below my shoulder blades. Perplexed, I look at the attending nurse and say,

"What's that I'm feeling on my back?"

"They are the connectors that can be used with a urine bag to catch your urine output if your kidneys fail. They are capped off right now because you don't need urine bags."

"I wasn't expecting this. I thought everything was going to be placed inside of me!"

"The nephrostomy tubes are inside of you. If your kidneys fail, however, we need a way to connect them to urine bags so you have the connectors (i.e., capsules)."

During my prior conversations with Dr. Aminu, when she spoke about the tubes being internalized, I didn't realize endpoints would be coming out of my body. I assumed the nephrostomy tubes would connect to my bladder or ureters or something, but nothing like this. So, this isn't what I was expecting.

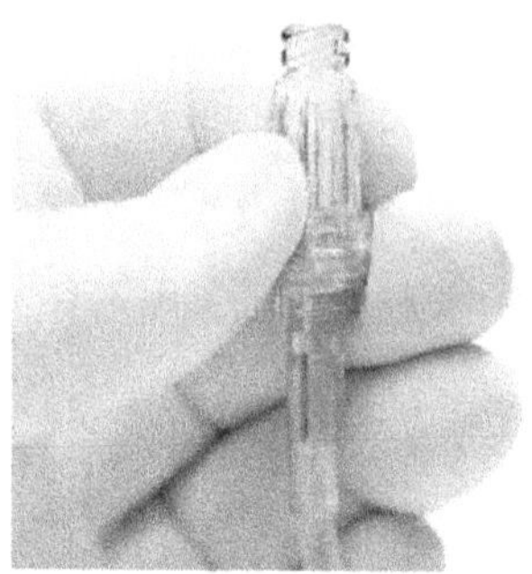

Nephrostomy Tube Needleness Connector

Now, I'm wondering how long these plastic capsules will be outside my body because they hurt like hell when I lie on my back, which is how I sleep. I'm not happy at all about this! Hopefully, I won't need the plastic "connectors" for very long. After the attending nurse wheels me back to my room, I call Bay to tell her the procedure went well. She's delighted to hear the news. When I tell her I have two stiff plastic capsules hanging out of my back and that they are very uncomfortable, she echoes my previous thought and says, "Well, hopefully, you won't have to have them very long." "I hope not," I reply.

Chapter 6
My New Reality

Today is Sunday, the fifth of December. These past nine days in the hospital have felt like an eternity! As I finish breakfast, Dr. Aminu stops by my room to see how I'm doing and informs me I'll be released from the hospital today at 2:00 P.M. "That's great! Thank you so much for trying to find out what is happening inside of me, I tell her." Before she leaves, she says she'll arrange for her office to schedule a follow-up visit with me within the next two weeks. "Okay," I say.

After Dr. Aminu leaves, I reflect on my hospital stay. My arms are purplish and adorned with needle pricks and bruises from all the blood tests I've undergone to check my PSA, creatinine levels, and kidney function. I haven't been able to sleep uninterrupted for nearly two weeks, as someone always needed more of my blood, had to change my urine bag or provide me with a status update. Returning home will be a huge relief, and I'm sure it will lift my spirits. Sleeping in a familiar bed should be helpful and allow me to get some much-needed rest. While there were some hiccups during my stay, like my seven-hour wait to have my nephrostomy tubes placed, most were attributable to COVID-19. It's been apparent the staff is emotionally, physically, and mentally drained from coping with the unfamiliar disease. However, Emory Healthcare's team, from janitors to receptionists, lab techs, nurses, and doctors, did an admirable job, especially considering COVID. So, I'm grateful for their efforts.

When Bay comes to pick me up, as we gather my belongings, a nurse comes into the room and says, "Mr. Simmons, when you're ready, I'll get your wheelchair to take you downstairs." I thank her and say, "We should be done in a few minutes." Following, she says, "Mrs. Simmons, if you want to bring your car to the hospital's front entrance, we'll meet you there." So, Bay and I kiss one another on the cheek, and she heads out to get the car. As the nurse wheels me out of my room, the other caretakers at the nurse's station wave me goodbye and say, "Good luck, Mr. Simmons." "Thank you all so much for taking great care of me," I tell them. Then I add, "As much as I'd like to come back and see you guys again, I'll do my best not to!" The nurses and some patients on the floor burst into laughter.

When the nurse and I get downstairs, Bay's already parked out front. She rolls the passenger window down, and the nurse tells her what a great patient I've been and that the hospital staff will miss me and my big smile. "Thank you and everyone involved for taking such good care of him," Bay expresses. "We're glad to be getting him back, however." as I embrace the nurse in a big hug to say goodbye, tears trickle down my face. I'm overwhelmed with emotions stemming from the bond I've formed with many of the hospital's staff members during my stay.

When we get home, Bay has a big surprise waiting for me. It's as if she has read my mind. She's readied the seldom used guest bedroom in the basement, so I don't risk falling down the wooden stairs connecting the house's second level, where the master and other bedrooms are located, to the main level. A beautiful new bedspread, sheets, and pillows are on the bed. An added benefit of my being in the basement is its full bathroom, so I can conveniently drain my urine bag. And I can also shower downstairs as long as I don't let the sutures in my back, from the placement of the nephrostomy tubes, get wet.

During my first few days at home, I do a ton of soul-searching. I have far more questions about my condition than there are answers. I'm asking myself, 'What could I have done to cause me to suffer like this? Whom have I wronged? What sin have I committed?' I'm also wondering why the doctors have so much difficulty finding out what's wrong with me. I could urinate, although painfully, before I went into the hospital, but once there, I couldn't. What happened? Did the cystoscopy exacerbate things and make matters worse? Is that what caused the complete blockage? Dr. Aminu says my prostate seems enlarged. So, do I have prostate cancer? I think I might. I've got tons of questions but no answers.

I finally realized I could worry myself to death trying to figure out all the what-ifs, whys, and how-comes. So, the best thing I can do is try to get better and trust the "bright light" I've seen. Plus, if I come unglued about my situation, so will Bay and the kids, so I must remain optimistic and trust that I will be all right for theirs and my mental well-being.

I'd been home about a week when K.J. walked in with a dog that looked just like Oreo, a pet of one of Pooh's co-workers that Pooh had cared for during the height of the pandemic. Unbeknownst to me, Bay, Pooh, and K.J. intended to adopt this "new" dog from a humane shelter and had "voted" to keep him without asking my opinion. Right off the bat, I was adamantly opposed to the idea because I was still recovering from my hospitalization and didn't feel I had the energy or patience for a pet. So, I told the trio that pets are like children, constantly requiring attention. And I also proclaimed, "I've already helped raise three children and am not ready for a fourth!" Conversely, the family thought the dog would benefit me from an exercise standpoint because I'd be getting out, walking, and building my strength. Still, having a dog right now was a bad idea, in my view.

After a few months, despite the dog pooping in the house several times, drinking water from the toilet, nearly biting me on one occasion, and falling asleep on the sofa in the family room - I could go on and on, I finally relented, and we adopted the dog. When it came time to name him, Bay wanted to go with Luca. I thought she was paying tribute to NBA All-Star Luka Dončić, but she told me the name was Jewish for bringer of light. I don't know if it was intentional on her part, but I immediately thought about the irony between the dog's name and the bright light that shone in my "room" in the ER. Forever the jokester, however, when I told Bay, "Well, we're the only Black family I know that has a dog with a Jewish name," we both chuckled.

One day, Luca and I are out walking, and we run into our next-door neighbors, Allah and Natoli, who are Jewish. When I tell them the dog's name, Allah says, "Oh, that's a nice name. It's Jewish for bringer of light." At that moment, I knew Luca was meant to be. But, as my neighbors walked off, I couldn't help but get tickled because I wondered if they were thinking, "Hmm, they're the only Black family we know that has a dog with a Jewish name."

And while I previously dreaded the prospect of keeping Luca, he's a walk in the park compared to the combination of my urine bag, catheter, sleeplessness, and nephrostomy tubes, which have all turned into an absolute nightmare! To begin with, before I left the hospital, a nurse showed me how to use Velcro straps to secure my urine bag to my leg so that I wouldn't have to carry the bag in my hand. However, my leg muscles expand and contract when I sit and stand, so the urine bag keeps slipping down my leg, and as a result, I'm constantly pulling down my pants to readjust the straps. Seeking a better solution, I've tried three or more options to secure the bag to my leg until I finally discovered that a leg bag works best for me. With it, I can wear it on the inside of either calf muscle and confidently go out in public without an embarrassing "bulge" in the thigh area of my pants. In addition, if the leg bag leaks, urine will stream down my socks or into or outside my shoes, which is a far better scenario than having a urine bag near my pelvic region because if it leaks, it will be evident I'd wet my pants.

Far from a "perfect" solution, however, my leg bag caused one of the most embarrassing moments of my life while I was shopping for groceries at Kroger one day. The device became so full and heavy with urine that it caused the tubing connected to the catheter to pull off. Subsequently, as I was nearing the store's doors to exit, urine began streaming onto the floor and making a trail with each of my steps out of the facility. Because there was nothing I could do to stop the urine flow, I was humiliated beyond words. Once outside the store, however, fortunately, a light rain started, so the urine stream from the bottom of my pant leg wasn't so noticeable as I walked through the parking lot to my car.

And my, oh my, my catheter. Imagine having a flexible plastic tube about the size of a pencil eraser and fourteen inches long running inside you from the head of your penis and into your bladder! And for good measure, the only time it can come out is when it needs to be changed every few months for sterility purposes. Then, at night, when you take your urine leg bag off, because it might leak while you're asleep and lying prone, you must attach the catheter to another urine bag, which in my case, can hold 4000 ml (i.e., about 9 pounds) of urine. The sturdy, barely pliable plastic tubing that connects the catheter to the more oversized urine bag is clear and about the roundness of a size AA battery but hollowed out. Imagine trying to sleep with this semi-hard piece of plastic across your thigh. It's like sleeping with a small "garden hose" across your leg.

At night, once I have the "larger" urine bag hooked to the bedrail on the left side, two things can happen when I lie down on my back. First, urine can flow onto the floor if the tube isn't secure on the urine bag's plastic male connector, and it accidentally pops off if I have turned to my right and begun urinating in my sleep. Second, urine will flow onto the bed if the tube happens to pop off its connector on the catheter near my penis. I've had both instances occur more times than I'd like to admit. And if that weren't enough, my nephrologist has me drinking 72 ounces of water daily, so I'm peeing a river at night. Wetting the bed and floor at my age

shames me and causes me to feel infantile. I have tried

sleeping on my stomach, but the catheter's "garden hose"

hose tube is too uncomfortable.

Also, my lack of sleep worries me immensely. Since I've

been home, I might get two hours of sleep a night. But,

many nights, I don't get any sleep. In addition to the urine

bag and catheter being culprits, another one is, I believe, my

Flomax medication, which, as I understand, is designed to

help me urinate. When I started taking Flomax, I noticed

that my back would itch like hell some nights. So, I would

call for Bay and ask her to come downstairs with a hairbrush

to "scratch" my back to help ease my discomfort. I

mentioned the itching to Dr. Aminu, but it was so sporadic

that it was hard to pinpoint it to the drug.

But, without a doubt, the most significant contributor to

my sleeplessness is these damn hard-assed nephrostomy

tubes! They are driving me insane. Several times I've

thought about trying to cut them off. I realize they're

necessary if my kidneys fail, but I didn't know I was getting

them in the first place! I've been told my kidneys must reach

a certain point of stability before the plastic couplings can be

removed, so I'm praying, like all get out, that my kidneys start

improving quickly! Some nights have been so bad due to the

nephrostomy tubes piercing my back and the seemingly

unending back itching that I've thought, 'If I had a gun handy, I would blow my brains out!' There've also been nights where I've thought about "accidentally" overdosing on my medication to make my death not look like a suicide! Before one of my follow-up visits, I had to fill out an online questionnaire. One of the questions was, "Have you had suicidal thoughts?" I only checked the "Yes" box because they didn't have one that said, "Hell Yeah!"

So, as I would lay crying in bed, I would ask, 'Lord, why are you putting me through this? You gave me a sign, in the form of a bright light, that everything would be all right. So, why must I suffer so?' Then, I would remind myself that there are people in this world who have it far worse than me, and if I were to commit suicide, the resultant psychological impact on my family would be devasting. So, I've got to fight. Dammit, I've got to fight through this pain and discomfort, even if it kills me!

So, I came up with a plan. At night, I started talking to the inside of my body. I would say to it, 'You've always been there for me. You've performed at a high level on big stages before, so please, I need you to do it again. Whatever's wrong with you, I need you to heal yourself. Attack whatever affects you now with a vengeance so I will be well again. I believe in you, so don't let me down now.' And as tears would roll down both of my cheeks, I would pray. "Dear

Lord, I apologize for my sins. I pray that you will look inside my heart. I believe the good I've done far outweighs the bad. So, I'll stop praying selfishly and asking you, 'Why me, Lord? Instead, I will say, Why not me, Lord? I'm no better than anyone else, so why not me, Lord? I know there's a reason why you have me going through this, but I don't know what it is. Maybe you're using me as an example because you want me to be a "light" for others. I don't know your reason why, but whatever it is, I accept it.' And so every time I would have a rough night with the plastic capsules and the itching, I would repeat this prayer.

Mercifully, my prayers and those of my family were being answered. By December 28th, my kidney function had improved drastically from a 6% GFR to stabilizing at 29% (i.e., Stage 4 Chronic Kidney Disease). Although I still wasn't out of the woods regarding my kidney function, the good news was that their functioning would have to drop nearly half for me to go back into the "dialysis range" (i.e., <15% GFR). And thankfully, on January 21st, 2022, Dr. Bellinger converted my nephrostomy tubes to indwelling ureteral stents. This step is what I had envisioned in the first place! Finally, my kidneys were stable enough that after fifty-three (53) torturous nights of pure hell, those hard-assed plastic capsules were removed! Now I could sleep on my back unimpeded by the two rigid synthetic vials! If I had been thinking, I should have asked Dr. Bellinger if I could keep the capsules, so I could take them home and hang them on my office wall as a reminder of what they put me through. But, no, I'm only kidding myself. I'd end up burning the damn things!

Chapter 7
Biopsy Test for Cancer

It's February 2nd, 2022, and I'm sitting in the lobby of Dr. Aminu's office. I'm thinking about the highs and lows I've been through the past two months and what a wild roller coaster of emotions it has been. It's been two weeks since the plastic "vials" on the end of my nephrostomy tubes were removed, and now I'm here to discuss the next steps of my medical care. To me, my current health situation seems unending. Plus, I'm already wondering if I have prostate cancer, and if I do, did she call this meeting to tell me such? And, as if to further heighten my anxiety, I'm scheduled to have another void trial today before I meet with Dr. Aminu. Again, the goal is to see if I can urinate without a catheter, which I know I can't, so I'm already sure I will fail the trial. So, today's news could end up being a double dose of disappointment.

A nurse escorts me into an exam room, and after about fifteen minutes of me trying to pee, I fail another void trial. After that, the attending nurse takes me to the opposite hallway and into a small room where Dr. Aminu's waiting and sitting in a chair, typing something into a computer. She stands to greet me and says, "Hello, Mr. Simmons. How are you doing today?" "Not so hot," I tell her. "Why is that?"

Dejectedly, I say, "Unfortunately, I failed another void trial." "Well, that's one of the reasons why I wanted to see you today," she says. "I'm still concerned about your enlarged prostate. So, I've scheduled you for a 3D MRI, CT Rectal exam, and prostate biopsy at our facility across town on the 14th of this month." When I ask, "Why across town?" she says, "Our facility there has one of the most advanced 3D MRIs in the state, and once your MRI and CT images are overlayed, they will give me an enhanced view of what's going on in your pelvic region and with your prostate. The biopsy will help me know if anything is happening with the cells in your prostate." I put my left hand over my mouth, shaking my head left and right as I go, "Unh-unh-unh."

After removing my hand, I ask, "The biopsy will reveal if I have cancer, correct?" It's a loaded question, and I already know Dr. Aminu can't answer it definitively yet, so I let her off the hook by continuing with, "I know you can't answer that." So, she replies, "I'm hoping it will give us a better idea of what's happening with you." After her comment, I sigh deeply, and my shoulders shake uncontrollably. As I start crying, I blurt out, "I can believe this. I'm a former athlete. Man, oh, man." After finally composing myself, I apologize to Dr. Aminu for my sudden outburst. "No worries, Mr. Simmons. When the imaging and biopsy results return, I'll schedule an appointment to bring you back to review the results," she says. All I can offer her is a disingenuous "Okay." On my way home, I'm in a moribund state, teared up and muttering, "Lord, please don't let me have cancer."

It's the morning of the 14th, the day of my appointment, and I'm listless, unfeeling, and numb from head to toe. I've reached a point regarding my healthcare situation where I no longer care. 'Satan's winning the battle, and I don't have the strength to fight back,' I think. My optimism and enthusiasm are at their lowest point since my hospitalization. It seems my "bright light" of hope has flickered out. Suddenly, I feel all alone.

I find an open space near the parking entrance when I get to the hospital. After parking and praying, as I walk across the lot to the hospital, I think, 'Well, this is it! The moment of truth has arrived. There's no turning back now. Soon my fate will reveal itself.' After checking in, a nurse comes and gets me to take me downstairs to the Radiology department. Once there, as we're walking down the hall, I look to my left, and there are four brand-spanking new CT scanners. Momentarily, I feel like a kid in a candy store. Memories of my days selling similar devices for GE's Medical Systems Division come flooding through, so I start a conversation with the nurse.

"I can't see the logo on the CT scanners. What brand are they?"

"Siemens. We just got them."

"Oh yes, it brings back memories. Probably our biggest competitor back in the day when I was selling diagnostic imaging equipment. Siemens makes good equipment."

"They sure do. Who did you use to work for?"

"GE Medical Systems."

"I was brought up on GE in nursing school, so they're still my favorite. When did you work for them?"

"A long time ago."

When we reach the end of the room where the CTs are located, we make a left turn, and the nurse takes me to a changing area to put on a hospital gown. Next, she shows me some combination lockers outside the changing rooms for storing my clothes and valuables. "When you finish changing, you can be seated in the waiting area, and someone will be with you shortly," she says. After putting on the hospital gown and storing my belongings, I return to the waiting area. A few minutes later, a nurse comes to get me and takes me into a room where I have to fill in some information on a computer. It includes my confirming I won't take jewelry or metal into the MRI area and also has the Hospital's disclaimer information - so they won't be sued. When I finish, the nurse takes me back to the waiting area.

About ten minutes later, a man in scrubs opens the door to my right, introduces himself, and tells me he's my MRI technician responsible for taking my images today. He leads me into a room with a new Siemens 3D MRI. As the tech sets up the unit to take pictures, I'm getting nervous because I'm aware the quality of MRI images is such that if I have cancer, the "mass" will show up. And when I factor in the 3D component, the tech will probably be the first to know if I have cancer.

My legs begin shaking while I'm sitting on the MRI's patient table, so the tech stops what he's doing, comes over to me, and says, "Don't worry. With today's technology, you're going to be okay. It just so happens I've got prostate cancer and am currently undergoing radiation treatment." "Really? Man, you look great," I tell him. "Thank you. I feel good. I'm one of five Black men in my church who currently have prostate cancer, and we're all in our fifties. So, we're supporting one another," he says. "That's great," I say. "I don't know why prostate cancer affects Black men more than other races." "Me either," he says. "But the good news is if you've got it, you're probably catching it early, and it can be treated. Let's hope you don't have it." "Amen to that," I proclaim!

As the tech has me lie down on the 3D MRI's patient table, he asks, "Are you claustrophobic?" I reply, "No, I'm not." "What type of music do you like?" he inquires, and I say, "R&B." Then he goes behind a glass window, fidgets with something, and comes back with headphones for me. When I put them on, he's got me jamming to the Whispers' "And the Beat Goes On." "Man, this is great," I tell him. Next, he goes back behind the glass window to what must be the MRI's control panel and says through the headphones, "Okay, Mr. Simmons, we're about to begin." After that, the patient table slowly moves me towards the machine's chamber. Once I'm inside the MRI, the headphones and music help mute the banging noise of the electromagnets when they turn off and on again.

I briefly stop humming to the music to see if I can recall how MRIs work. Let's see now, 'When the magnets turn on, the hydrogen atoms in my body will come to an erect state. When turned off, the particles wobble and emit electrical signals captured by sensors in the magnet's shell that get sent to a computer that uses mathematical formulas to convert that data into images. How did someone figure this stuff out?' Then I snap out of trying to remember how these incredible machines work and revert to listening to the music coming from my headphones. The tunes are so soothing that I fall asleep inside the magnet. I finally wake up when the patient table begins rolling me out of the 3D imager.

After the table stops, the tech comes out from where he was taking the images, and I ask, "How long was I in there? I fell asleep." "About forty minutes," he says. Curious, I ask how the images look, knowing he can't tell me. "Mr. Simmons, I'm not allowed to divulge that information. It has to come from your doctor." "I know it does, and my apologies for putting you on the spot. I'm just anxious to find out if I have cancer so I can begin trying to prepare myself mentally," I divulge. "No worries. I understand," he says. After that, he takes me back to the waiting area, where we wish one another well as he departs.

I'm checking my cellphone for messages when a nurse comes to get me to take me to the room where I'm to have my biopsy and CT Rectal exam. When we arrive, she introduces me to Dr. Rossi, a urologist, who tells me she will perform both procedures. As we chat, I find Dr. Rossi's bedside manner cordial to the extent that I'm beginning to trust her. So, with my hands sweating on the padded-covered table I'm sitting on, I disclose how nervous I am about the biopsy and CT Rectal exam. As she's reassuring me neither procedure will be that bad, I'm starting to feel pretty good about them until she says, "I'll be performing the biopsy through your anus." It had never dawned on me that the biopsy would be done that way. Not looking forward to my butt receiving any more attention than it already has and is about to, I try to make light of my situation. I quip, "After this, I will have broken the Guinness World Record for the most fingers and probes up one butt in four months!" After that, she and the nurse chuckle.

Next, Dr. Rossi had me lie on my stomach for the CT Rectal exam. As she begins performing the exam, I ask her if the probe I feel going up my anus is the camera, and she says, "Yes, it is." "This exam isn't bad at all," I tell her. After Dr. Rossi finishes the "procedure," I'm given a five-minute break before the biopsy begins. While I'm resting, she and the nurse are preparing for the biopsy. When they finish, Dr. Rossi says, "Okay, Mr. Simmons, I'm about to begin the biopsy. First, I'll numb the area and then use a device to take twelve samples from your prostate. As I take each fragment, you'll hear a clicking sound go off like a staple gun; then, you'll feel a pinch. So, I want you to count from one to ten to help you relax as I take each sample. Now, I'll need you to lie on your left side, pull your legs towards me, and get in a semi-fetal position." After I do, I feel a small tube going up my anus, followed by a cool sensation, so I ask Dr. Rossi if what I'm feeling is something to numb the area of my prostate, and she tells me it is. "Now, we must wait a few minutes while the numbing takes effect." So, after a few minutes pass, she says, "Okay, I'm about to take the first sample. Remember now, count from one to ten for me. You can start now." So, I start counting, "One, two, three, four," and when the staple gun goes off, I feel a sharp snip that feels like someone has taken some tweezers and quickly pulled the skin off the inside my prostate. That shit hurt!

I can feel Dr. Rossi moving to different locations inside my prostate as she takes the second and third samples, and with each one, I'm experiencing increasing anxiety and discomfort. I think a lot of it relates to the echoing in the room each time the stapler goes off. First, I cringe because it sounds like I'm being shot at, and then, in my mind, it feels like a large chunk of my prostate is being removed versus a small piece. So as Dr. Rossi's about to take the fourth fragment, I count, "One, two, three, ten!" I've already had enough of this biopsy business, and getting to twelve samples seems light-years away! Finally, noticing I'm mentally ready to throw in the towel, Dr. Rossi says, "Try to think about something pleasant as I take the samples. That should help ease the discomfort a bit." I want to say, 'The only enjoyable thing I can think of right now is getting the hell out of here,' but I don't.

As sample after sample is being taken out, I've become so mentally numb that Dr. Rossi could take out my entire prostate for all I care. At last, finally, the twelfth sample is taken. After that, I breathe a long sigh of relief. I want to say out loud, "If I hadn't stopped drinking six years ago, I could use a cold Bud Lite right about now!" Now that both procedures are done, and I've gotten my faculties together, I say goodbye to Dr. Rossi before she departs. Next, the nurse escorts me back to the locker where my clothes are stored. After I get dressed, she walks me to the exit to the hospital's lobby. As I walk through the open area, I wonder if people are thinking, 'Gee, that guy is walking like he has a stick up his ass.' If that is what they are wondering, little do they know it feels like I do.

Chapter 8
Prostate Cancer Confirmed

More convinced than ever that I have prostate cancer, I looked into treatment options before my appointment with Dr. Aminu to discuss my rectal exam and biopsy results. I want to be as prepared and knowledgeable as possible when I meet with her and be able to express my preferred course of treatment. Getting ahead of the curve and having a say in my treatment plan is, to me, very important. If I have prostate cancer and can avoid undergoing radiation or chemotherapy treatment, I prefer having my prostate removed via the least invasive surgery possible. So, given my fascination with technology and experience in medical sales, I researched to see if technology was available to remove a prostate robotically. A robot's precision cutting capability, I feel, will be far better than having two, possibly "large" human hands inside me. So, over the weekend, using Google's search engine, I found two YouTube videos on "mechanized prostate removal" that intrigue me. Viewing the videos, I discover that a robotic-assisted prostatectomy is the surgical removal of a prostate using a robot. Watching the procedure, I'm blown away by the technology and its use.

While viewing the videos, my misconception that a robot would primarily control the surgical procedure is incorrect.

Instead, a doctor operates using equipment such as a high-powered surgical light, cameras, monitors, an articulated robotic arm(s)/hand(s), scalpel-like tools, etc. So as the doctor performs the surgery with his hands, the robot mimics the surgeon's every move and subsequently executes the procedure, which I find amazing! And, because a robot's hands can be manufactured to be smaller than a human's, the surgery is much less invasive, which appeals to me. I'll take the tiny "appendages" of a robot over "large" hands being inside me any day! So, I plan to let Dr. Aminu know that if I have prostate cancer, and if at all possible, I want to have a robotic-assisted prostatectomy done. Therefore, my million-dollar question is, "Does Emory Healthcare offer it?" If not, I'll try to see if I can get into the Mayo Clinic or another high-profile cancer treatment center that does.

I've been checking MyChart, Emory Healthcare's "patient portal," for my biopsy results for two days, and nothing has been posted. Finally, the results are posted on the third day of checking. Before opening the Clinical Notes, I pray, "Lord, please don't let me have cancer." When I open the notes, there are a lot of medical terms I don't understand, but I can somewhat make out some of the information, which is alphabetized. Section A shows I have a Gleason score of 7, which I suspect isn't good. It also says, "Gleason pattern 4 comprising 80% of the tumor. Perineural invasion identified." So, I have a tumor, but I can't tell from what I'm reading if it's cancerous or not. The information also appears to be saying something has leaked out to the outer membrane of my prostate; at least, that's how I'm interpreting it. Sections B through D show benign prostatic glands and stroma, so I may not have prostate cancer after all. Oh, no! Sections E, F, and G all show prostatic adenocarcinoma. I'm not a doctor, and I don't need a Google search to tell me, but when I see the words tumor and carcinoma, I know it means I've got cancer. Man, oh man, I'm screwed!

Tears roll down my face as what I've just read in the Clinical Notes begins to soak in. I'm heartbroken to the extent; I can't bear to read the rest of the report. I have mixed feelings about discovering that I have prostate cancer before my doctor has had a chance to tell me. On the one hand, I wish I'd never opened the Clinical Notes and regret that I did. But on the other hand, I may have gone mad waiting the two weeks when I'm scheduled to meet with Dr. Aminu for her to review my biopsy results.

Bay, Pooh, and Kevin are upstairs, so it takes me about ten minutes to compose myself before I can muster up the courage to break the news to them. I'll text Dee right after I speak with the others. Once upstairs with the three, I say, "The biopsy results are back. While I still have to wait for confirmation from Dr. Aminu, the report shows I have cancer in my prostate." Right after my disclosure, Bay rocks back on her heels, and her eyes roll up in her head, but she doesn't faint. K.J. and Pooh are standing with their mouths open, speechless. When I ask them to pray that my cancer is treatable, Bay says, "I'm already claiming you're going to beat your cancer!" After Bay's declaration, the kids and I say, "We're claiming it too!" When I text Dee, to my surprise, he doesn't come unglued, as I had expected. Instead, he replies, "Don't worry, Dad. God's got this!"

So, two weeks pass, and I'm at Dr. Aminu's office to discuss my rectal exam and biopsy results. Before I meet with her, and to my dismay, she's scheduled me for what I'm sure will be another futile void trial attempt. The test will be at least my fourth attempt to urinate without a catheter. And each time previously, I've gone in highly optimistic, but after I fail the procedure, I leave utterly devasted. So, I'm frustrated about what I feel is an unnecessary step. After a nurse escorts me to an exam room for the trial, this time, like my last two attempts, when I try to pee, there's a red-hot pain so intense that I drop to my knees while maybe one or two drops of urine come out. However, this time, I am not as bummed out about my failure as in the past because I knew I would fail the test. I guess this was Dr. Aminu's last "Hail Mary" attempt.

Following my failed void trial, I told the attending nurse I'd decided over the weekend to finally give self-catheterizing a try because I was sick and tired of wearing a leg bag. During my last two office visits, when I was asked to think about self-catheterizing, each time, I declined because **psychologically, I couldn't** bear the thought of sticking a fourteen (14) inch catheter up my penis and into my bladder. So, surprised by my change of heart, the nurse tells me she's confident I'll be able to successfully self-catheterize. Following, she goes and gets a catheter, puts some gloves on, takes it out of its packaging, hands it to me, and exits the exam room.

As I'm painstakingly pushing the catheter up my penis, I think, 'This is total madness! Something's supposed to come out of, not go up into one's penis.' After several attempts, I'm so uptight about having this long plastic tube in my penis that when I finally reach my sphincter muscle which relaxes and closes to allow urine to flow and stop from the bladder, it feels like I've hit a brick wall. It's as if the tendon is saying, 'Look, try as you might, but I'm not opening my door and letting that damn catheter get past me!' So, I try to relax and push more firmly, but when I do, it feels like I've slightly torn my sphincter. When I glance down at the catheter, the small green triangle, used as a visual to ensure the device is lined up correctly, isn't straight. Instead, it's turned to the right. So, while in some pain, I slowly back the catheter out, and sure enough, there's blood on its tip. Thinking I've nicked my sphincter muscle, I open the door and call for the nurse. When she returns to the exam room, I tell her how far I made it and about the subsequent blood on the tip of the catheter. Having failed at self-catheterizing, I ask the nurse to insert a new catheter in me, and she does.

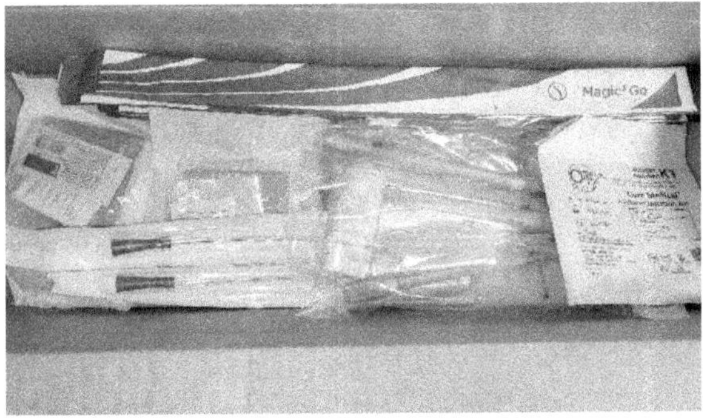

Box of catheter supplies

After I get dressed, the nurse takes me to another examination room where Dr. Aminu awaits. After we greet one another, I tell her about my failed void trial and self-catheterization attempt. She says not to worry and that I'll eventually be able to self-catheterize. My heart sinks as I settle into my chair, knowing she's about to confirm I have prostate cancer. I lean forward, my hands holding onto my chair's armrests like vise grips. I'm dreading what she's about to tell me and its severity. I'm also wondering how my cancer will affect my lifespan.

Dr. Aminu begins by telling me she's reviewed my 3D MRI, CT Rectal exam, and biopsy. Next, she says, "Your biopsy revealed cancer in forty percent (40%) of your prostate." I thought I'd be ready for the confirmation of my prostate cancer, but I'm far from it. My head drops; I shake it left, right, and left, and go, "Unh, unh, unh." Then, I take a deep breath, exhale, and say, "Whew!" After that, I ask Dr. Aminu, "How long do I have to live?" I already know she can't answer the question. She pauses, then says, "I'm sorry, I don't know. All I can tell you is that you are in a bad way, and we must act fast."

So, before Dr. Aminu begins to lay out my treatment options, I tell her about my research on robotic prostate surgery and ask, "Does Emory Healthcare offer it?" She immediately replies, "Yes, we do, and we're one of the best at it!" I perk up and say, "That's great! I want the robot!" "Well," she says, "Why don't we review all your treatment options first?" Unfortunately, while Dr. Aminu's laying out three options for my treatment, I'm only partially listening because my mind is focused on robotic surgery. When I realize I could be missing something vital that she's saying, I interrupt, saying, "My apologies; I guess I'm a little shaken about today's news, and I'm only half listening. Would you mind starting over?" "It's understandable, and I don't mind at all," she says. "You have three options based on what we currently know about your situation. One, we can do "active surveillance" of your prostate to see if your condition worsens. Second, you could undergo hormone treatment with radiation. Third, you could have a robotic prostatectomy, which might be complemented with hormone treatment and radiation if cancer has spread outside your prostate." Before Dr. Aminu can hardly finish her last sentence, nearly shouting, I say, "I want the robot!" Following, she says, "However, I need to collaborate with my peers first because your situation is unique and quite complex. You've got a lot going on with your prostate. So, I'll set up another meeting with you in two weeks. We'll probably meet at the location where you had your MRI." "Okay. I'll watch MyChart for the date," I tell her.

When I get home, I update Bay and the kids on my meeting with Dr. Aminu. "It's confirmed. I have prostate cancer," I tell them. As my news is sinking in, I also let them know I've requested robotic surgery to remove my prostate, and Emory Healthcare offers it and is one of the best at it. "That's great," Bay says. "Do you know when you'll be having the procedure?" "I don't know yet. Dr. Aminu wants to brainstorm with some of her peers because she says my situation is unique and complex. So, I'll learn more about the surgery's timeframe after I meet with her in two weeks. She's pretty young, and while I believe she can do the surgery, considering the uniqueness of my situation, I prefer someone more seasoned. So, I'll go onto Emory Healthcare's website and read up on their urologists who have a good amount of experience performing robotic prostate removal."

"For now, I'm only telling each of you, Dee, a few family members, and maybe a couple of close friends, that I have prostate cancer. As well-intentioned as they might be, I don't need people bugging me right now and asking me a million questions, thinking they are a doctor, and telling me I can cure my prostate cancer by soaking my feet in beetle juice or something ludicrous like that. And there'll be those telling me they know other men with prostate cancer, and they're doing fine. But cancer behaves differently in each person, and my situation is further complicated because I've got an issue with my kidneys. So, I'm definitely outside the "norm" in that regard. And if it's true that 55% of the people you befriend don't feel the same way as you (according to averages in a PLOS ONE article), Lord knows I don't want the "gossipers" to get wind of this. They probably wish me dead anyway. Or by the time they finished spreading rumors, cancer would have caused me to have grown a tail, so No to their nonsense! I'll let them know on my terms and when I'm healed!" After finishing my sermon, Bay's eyes are so glazed over that I hurry downstairs to search for Emory Healthcare

prostate cancer surgeons to identify the one I'd like to

request.

Chapter 9
Prostate Cancer Loves Bones

From the moment I discovered in the "Clinical Notes" I have prostate cancer to Dr. Aminu's confirmation, I believe I should be proactive regarding my cancer. While I appreciate my doctors giving me their medical advice and opinions, it's critical that I "own" my situation because it's my life at stake, not theirs. So this ownership, I feel, involves me researching prostate cancer and educating myself on treatment plans. I want to feel comfortable asking my doctors tough questions and be in a position of intelligently versus emotionally challenging them if I disagree on something or need clarification. At the same time, I suspect I don't have much time to overanalyze things and spend my time and energy on dozens of second opinions. Since my cancer has already consumed forty percent of my prostate and appears to be growing, I need to be as decisive in my decision-making as possible and reach out to others, if need be, for help.

So, the day after my prostate cancer was confirmed, I called Dr. Linda Cunningham (nee Fairries), my old high school girlfriend. We only dated for about a month because I "chickened out," which is another story. I first met Linda during our ninth-grade year in junior high and developed a massive crush on her. But when I had mustered up enough courage to try to date her, one of my best friends and basketball teammate, Anthony Sharpe, made me aware that he had just started dating her. Back then, we basketball players had an unwritten rule - never talk to (i.e., try to date) one of your teammates' or friends' girlfriends, so Linda was "off limits" as far as our basketball "code" of ethics went. I was also friends with her sister Andrea through her dating my friend Jerome Liggett, and it was through their relationship I met Mr. and Mrs. Fairries, Linda and Andrea's parents. So, I've been a friend of the family for years.

After graduating high school, Linda attended the University of Alabama and, following her graduation, was accepted to Vanderbilt's School of Medicine, where she received her doctorate. Aside from Bay and the kids, Linda would be the first person I would tell I have cancer. My reason for reaching out to her, albeit reluctantly, is to see if she wouldn't mind being my "medical mentor" to help me navigate the medical "undercurrent" I feel I'll be in for a while. I don't want to drown, so to speak, from a lack of understanding of medical terminology, procedures, prescription side effects, etc. So, I need someone to serve as a "lifeline" to help guide me through this murkiness called prostate cancer. However, I'm reluctant to ask her for help because her husband, Henry, also an MD, had passed away from colon cancer. Aware of her pain with his passing, I don't know if she can cope with assisting a friend right now with their cancer. But I'm willing to risk asking for her help because I want someone other than my current doctors to provide me with not necessarily a second opinion but advice, insight, and guidance during this rough patch. Linda will shoot straight with me and provide unfiltered information about my medical condition. And, if I need to get my will in order, she won't pull any punches when telling me. Also, I might have to have another shoulder to cry on occasionally, and I don't think she'll mind.

During my call with Linda, when I tell her I've been diagnosed with prostate cancer and it's in forty percent of my prostate, she tells me her medical discipline is pathology (the study of the causes and nature of diseases). She says one of her duties is the analysis of prostate biopsies and presenting her findings to attending physicians. I'm floored to learn this! So, when I ask her if she wouldn't mind being my "medical mentor," without hesitating, she says, "But of course!" Hearing this news, I thank her and tell her how thrilled I am that she is willing to be there for me. After we hang up, I can't help but think, 'What are the odds that my old high school girlfriend is a pathologist specializing in diseases like prostate cancer? What a Godsend!'

Later that night, I confide to Bay, "As strange as it may seem, I'm relieved my doctors have finally discovered what's happening with me. Not knowing these past few months has been driving me nuts. At least now I know what's occurring inside me, and my doctors can develop a treatment plan." I don't tell her about my constant wondering whether I will live or die. However, I tell her I am more worried about my kidneys failing and possibly being placed on dialysis than I am concerned about my prostate cancer. She encourages me not to worry and **tells me** I need to continue drinking plenty of water, as my nephrologist (i.e., kidney doctor, as I call the folks) has prescribed, and be sure I do everything he asks me. I assure her I will.

Unfortunately, my relief to finally learn what is happening with my body is short-lived. A few weeks later, during a follow-up visit with Dr. Aminu, she made me aware prostate cancer likes to attack bones, and as a result, she wants me to have a "full nuclear body scan" right away to see if the cancer has invaded my bones. I'm both stunned and devasted by the news. I think, 'If cancer has started attacking my bones, I'm as good as dead.' For some reason, I've always equated bone cancer with imminent death, so I'm viewing a nuclear body scan as the deliverer of that message.

On my way home, I can't help but break down crying. Since my hospitalization, it seems every time I get good news, bad news follows, and now the prospect that I might have bone cancer is more than I can bear. I feel I'm a dead man if cancer has invaded my bones. This news is the worst information I could have received right now. So, when I get home, and after the garage door closes, I stay in my car for a minute to wipe my eyes and regroup before going inside to give Bay the news. After telling her about my upcoming nuclear scan, I can see she's very concerned, so to lift her spirits, I say, "Don't worry, Bay, I'll be fine. It's just a precautionary measure." What I don't tell her is that I'm scared shitless. My state of mind has turned me into a complete hypocrite because I'm reneging on my promise to God. Instead of saying, 'Why not me, Lord?' All I can think of is, 'Why me, Lord?'

On the morning of my nuclear body scan, I'm lethargic and have practically given up on life. When Bay asks me how I feel, I say, "Not so good." So she tries to cheer me up, but I'm in no mood, so I brush her off. Then, aware of my rudeness, I give her a half-hearted apology before she heads to work. After I get to the hospital, a nurse takes me into a room with a nuclear scanner. While she prepares me for the scan, I ask her how long it will take, and she says, "About forty-five minutes to an hour." Next, I ask, "When will I get the results?" "Usually in a few days, but it could be sooner. COVID has everything backed up right now," she says. I utter, "I can only imagine."

As I'm sitting on the patient table of the scanner, I'm scared to death. Soon, the nurse has me lie on my back, and as the scanner's table slowly moves me towards its chamber, I'm praying that cancer hasn't spread to my bones. I feel isolated and alone in the doughnut-shaped structure as it whirs, and the table slowly jerks each time a section of my body is scanned. 'Do I need to get my will updated? Are all my affairs in order so Bay and the kids won't struggle to find important information if I die? What will it be like for them once I'm gone?' These thoughts and more are going through my mind when suddenly the scanner stops. Then, the table starts moving me out of its cylinder. Thinking the first part of the scan is complete and I'll have to wait to be rescanned, the nurse says, 'That's it. You're done.' Stunned, I say, "You're kidding! It seems like I was only in there for about thirty minutes." "You were. Now, I've got to talk to the radiologist," she says.

So, the nurse leaves and walks into a room with a large rectangular window where a man wearing a white coat is sitting. I'm assuming he's the radiologist and is reviewing the scan. Watching the two chat, I nervously think, 'I was in and out of the scanner so fast; he must have seen cancer in my bones and concluded there was no need to scan further.' So, now, I'm sick to my stomach. When the nurse returns, I try pumping her for information about the scan results, knowing she can't tell me due to hospital protocol. So, as I expect, she says, "Your doctor has to be the one to share with you your test results." Undaunted, I press her for information until she doesn't break but bends slightly. Finally, cautiously and almost cryptically, she says, "Mr. Simmons, the fact that the doctor is sending you home early…." Then she stops talking. I can read between the lines, though, and what she's telling me with her "code-speak" is, 'Further testing isn't necessary because you're in the clear!' Tears well up in my eyes; I reach over, hug her, and thank the Lord. Sure enough, the next day, my results in MyChart show I've tested negative for cancer in my bones. I throw my hands in the air and yell, Hallelujah! Then, I run upstairs to tell Bay the great news.

Chapter 10
My Treatment Options

With hospital staff and patients required to wear masks due to COVID, I'm not sure, but Dr. Aminu seems pretty young to me, so when I do a Google search on her, Emory Healthcare's website show she's less than two years removed from medical school. Considering I have a "unique" situation, as she previously put it, and with no offense to her, if I can have robotic surgery, I prefer someone with much more experience. So in preparation for my March meeting with her to review my prostate cancer treatment options, I have identified three Emory Healthcare urologists with more experience than her that I'd prefer to perform my surgery. Also anticipating that I might require hormone therapy, I've found three of the Healthcare system's oncologists specializing in cancer treatment.

I compiled multiple names because I want alternatives if a doctor I'm interested in isn't available. I've also created a PowerPoint slide on which, on the right side, I've typed the names of the six physicians I've found. After that, I Googled "color image of a prostate" and "color image of an enlarged prostate." I've located two pictures I like and copied and pasted them onto the slide. As a visual learner, the pictures and other information I'm compiling are helpful because they help me better understand what has happened to me. I also want to converse with Dr. Aminu intelligently about why I find robotic surgery and hormone treatment preferable. I believe having the final say about my medical care is incumbent upon me. However, I realize my seeking another urologist is risky because I might offend Dr. Aminu. If she disagrees with me and feels she should perform the procedure, I'll have to put my foot down and tell her that if I can't get whom I want for the surgery, I'll have to look at the Mayo Clinic or elsewhere.

Since I've never had a health "crisis" like this before, I've never had to tell a doctor I prefer someone else. So my upcoming meeting with Dr. Aminu could get pretty testy. While my desire for another urologist might offend her, I'm willing to take the risk because my life is on the line here. As a result, I want the most seasoned and experienced physician I can get to perform my surgery. The day after I'd completed my PowerPoint slide, I received an email informing me I had a new appointment in MyChart. Upon checking, Dr. Aminu has scheduled my treatment plan meeting with her for March 6th.

Before leaving the house On the morning of the 6th for my appointment with Dr. Aminu, I print two copies of my PowerPoint slide, one with my chosen doctors' names and one without them. I plan to give her the latter. I put the material in a glossy Emory Healthcare folder to not give away my intentions and into one of Pooh's old college volleyball backpacks. On my drive to the hospital, I can't help but wonder how Dr. Aminu's going to react to my request for another surgeon. Per MyChart, our appointment is at the Winship Cancer Institute of Emory University. I'm to park in the Purple lot, which is free for cancer patients, and located across from the facility. While I understand the need for easy access parking for cancer patients and appreciate that it's free, having "special" parking makes me feel somewhat like I'm now viewed as "handicapped."

When I check in at the ground floor level of the Cancer Institute, a receptionist directs me to the Hematology and Medical Oncology department on the first floor. Once there, after about a five-minute wait, a nurse comes to get me. She takes me into an exam room, checks my vitals, tells me they all look good, and when she's finished, says, "Dr. Aminu will be with you shortly." After the nurse leaves, I pull the folder from Pooh's backpack and lay it on my lap. I'm fidgeting a little, so to calm my nerves and take my mind off my impending conversation, I pull up the ESPN app on my phone to catch up on the latest sports news. After a few minutes, there's a knock on the door, and after I say, "Come in," in walks Dr. Aminu. When I stand up, I nearly drop my folder, and as we shake hands, she says, "Mr. Simmons, how are you doing today?" "A little nervous," I reply. "That's understandable," she says. "But, before we begin, I'd like to give you a rectal exam to see if your prostate has continued to enlarge." After I mutter, "Okay," I drop my pants and underwear and lean over on an exam table, saying to myself 'I sure as hell hope she doesn't know what I'm about to discuss with her. If so, she'll probably shove her finger through my rear up to my throat during the exam.' The rectal exam starts well, and I feel no significant discomfort. Then, without warning, Dr. Aminu's finger goes higher into my anus, and when it touches my prostate, it feels like her whole fist is inside me. Yep, she knows I'm requesting another doctor, and she's pissed! After Dr. Aminu finishes the exam, I exhale loudly, "Whew!"

I pull up my underwear and pants and gingerly take a seat. Dr. Aminu is sitting across from me in front of a computer on my right. She asks me if I have any questions, and I say, "Yes, lots of them. But before we get started, I'd like to share something with you. Being a visual learner, I put together several prostate images on a PowerPoint slide to help me better understand what I think has happened to me. So, I'd like to share what I believe has occurred." Dr. Aminu nods her head in approval and replies, "Sure." I pull out both slides, printed on 8 1/2 by 11 paper, and hand one to her. Looking down at my copy, I realize I've given her the one with the names on it! 'Dammit! I'm busted! Now she knows I'm looking for physician resources other than her. Since it's out there now, I might as well proceed.'

I begin with, "As I understand, my prostate has enlarged due to cancer growing inside it. Over time, the tumor has grown, causing my prostate to swell internally and push against my urethra, rendering it almost entirely shut. With nowhere to go, urine has collected in my bladder, thus causing toxicity in my kidneys and resulting in them nearly failing. Quite honestly, I'm surprised my bladder didn't rupture or burst. As my bladder expanded, it pushed my stomach up into my sternum. Now, with my stomach being so "scrunched up," that caused me to lose my appetite and become malnourished. And that explains why I've lost so much weight. Is that about, right? If not, please explain to me, in layperson's terms, what's been going on with my body."

Eric Simmons

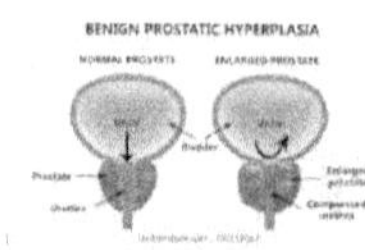

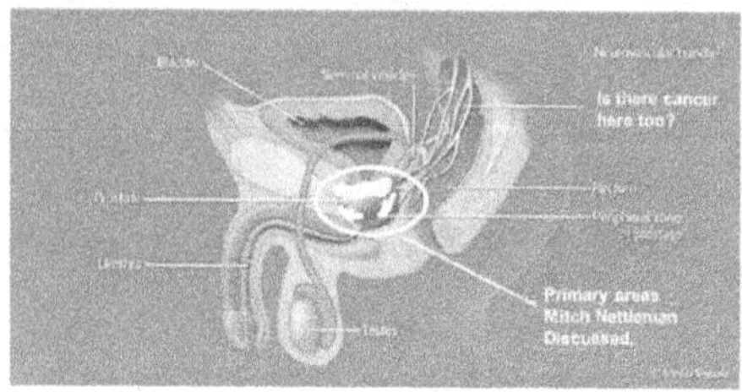

PowerPoint I prepared for a discussion with my urologist.

Dr. Aminu clears her throat and says, "Well, Mr. Simmons. First, imagine the male prostate as an orange. Next, envision the urethra, the tube that allows urine to flow through the penis, being a straw going through the middle of the orange. As your cancer cells grew inside the orange, pressure began to be applied to the "straw," which ultimately became shut. So, when your "straw" became shut, urine began to back up into your bladder, which became so large, and you're correct, that your stomach reached your sternum. Then, as your bladder became full, your kidneys became overloaded and swelled because urine wasn't being expelled". "That makes total sense," I say. Next, as she peruses the handout I hadn't intended to give her, I can tell she's scanning the names on it. The room is so quiet you can hear a mouse peeing on cotton. I'm getting nervous and thinking, 'Oh, boy, here it comes. She's going to blow a gasket, then I'll blow mine, and it will get ugly up in here real quick!'

To my astonishment, she says, "You know, Mr. Simmons. I've been thinking. Because your situation is unique, I'd like to refer you to someone with more experience than I have, if that's okay with you. The names on your list are good, but I don't know the doctors' availability. And because I'd like to get you into surgery as soon as possible, I have someone else in mind. I'm thinking about my boss, Dr. Sharp." I'm so stunned by what I've just heard; my mouth drops open, and I'm speechless, which is impossible for someone as talkative as me. Fortunately, Dr. Aminu and I aren't going to have a confrontation after all. As it turns out, my fears were completely unfounded, and we're both on the same page. I can't believe it! What a relief!

When I'm finally able to speak, I say, "I was worried you might take my research the wrong way, and I would end up offending you." "No worries, Mr. Simmons. I think someone with more experience is best for you," she replies. Then, like an idiot, I say, "So, Dr. Sharp's pretty good, huh?" Next, she hits me with a zinger I deserve. "I wouldn't recommend him if he weren't," she asserts. "But the problem is that he only performs surgeries on Tuesdays and Thursdays, so I don't know if he'll be available in the timeframe I'd like you to have your procedure. So, I'll have to check with him about his schedule." "If he's available, I'd like to request him, but with one condition," I state. "I want you in there assisting him. Since it seems my surgery will be complex, I believe the experience will benefit you in your future surgeries." "I agree," she says, "and I'll do my best to be there. "Within the next few days, I'll let you know if my boss is available."

Dr. Aminu and I stand and shake hands before she heads out for her next appointment. After she leaves, I let out a big sigh of relief while putting my folder back into the backpack. As I head out, just before I reach the exit door, I hear "Mr. Simmons. Oh, Mr. Simmons." When I turn around, Dr. Aminu's in a semi-jog and coming up the hall. She catches up with me and says, "I just ran into my boss, and he says he'll do your surgery." Thrilled, I say, "That's great news!" Next, she says, "I've got an appointment right now, so if you would, please see our scheduler, who's just around the corner, and tell him I want you on my boss's calendar for a pre-surgery meeting." I thank Dr. Aminu, and after she leaves, I walk around the corner of the exam area and introduce myself to the scheduler.

"Hello, I'm Eric Simmons," I say to the scheduler. "Dr. Aminu wants me to get on Dr. Sharp's schedule this month for a pre-prostate surgery meeting." "Okay, let me pull up his calendar," the scheduler says. While he does so, wanting further confirmation of Dr. Sharp's skills, I say, "I hope he's as good as Dr. Aminu says." After that, the scheduler clears his throat, tugs on his N95 mask, sternly looks at me, and says, "He's the best!" Still unsure, I remark, "He's that good?" The scheduler, now appearing offended, cocks his head to the side, looks me in the eyes, and says, "If it were me, my father, or one of my relatives needing prostate surgery, I would want Dr. Sharp to do it. People worldwide come to see this man for prostate surgery, so you're lucky you could get him." Then he nods at me as if to say in the words of Biggie Smalls, "If you didn't know, now you know!" "Wow, that's fantastic! Thank you so much for sharing that with me. I feel so much better now," I reply. "There, you're on his calendar," the scheduler says. "You'll see it in MyChart when you get home."

Wanting to know more about Dr. Sharp, I Googled him when I got home and found his credentials most impressive. I'm thrilled and relieved to get someone as experienced and talented as he to perform my surgery. I can't wait to share my good news with Bay when she gets home. When she does, I first tell her about my meeting with Dr. Aminu and that she recommends someone with more experience than she performs the surgery. Then I add, "It turns out her boss, who's world-renowned, has agreed to do it." Bay smiles and says, "See, I told you everything would work out." Next, I confess again and say, "Bay, I'm still much more worried about my kidneys than my prostate cancer because I believe I'll beat my cancer. The bright light I saw has already made it so. But man, oh man, if my kidneys fail, I don't know what'll happen next. I don't want to be on dialysis for the rest of my life." To ease my concerns, Bay says, "Well, your kidneys are improving, and if you keep drinking plenty of water and listen to your doctor, I believe you'll be okay. We both need to look into foods that are good for the kidneys. I'll do some research and want you to do some too." "Okay," I tell her.

Later in the evening, I call Linda with an update, but she doesn't answer, so I leave her a voicemail. A few days pass, and she calls me back, apologizing for missing my call. She says, "Hi there, I'm in Jerusalem on vacation, but I got your voicemail and wanted to get back to you." When I tell her it could have waited until she returned to the States, she replies, "Oh, no, I want you to keep me updated. From what you've told me, I can tell that you're in good hands with the folks at Emory Healthcare. You're a good patient, and you take the time to research to pose intelligent questions to your doctors. You have always been inquisitive and should want to know what's happening with your body. But unfortunately, many patients don't ask questions. So, keep asking questions, and feel free to call me if there's something you don't understand." "Thank you again for being so accommodating and making yourself available. I appreciate it more than you'll ever know," I tell her.

Then she says, "Butch, there's one thing I don't want you to do, and that is to sit around feeling sorry for yourself. It would be best if you keep your everyday routine. Get out, have fun, and enjoy life. So now that I think about it, you and Bay should schedule a vacation and come to Jerusalem. She'd love it, and you would too." When I remind Linda about Bay's work schedule, she replies, "Well then, get over here when you can." "If I had your money," I reply, "I would." Then, she fires back with, "Who says I have money? I'm retired now. I worked hard for forty years. I've decided that now it's time for me to spend time on me, and you and Bay should do the same." When I reply, "Point taken," she says, "I'll call you when I return to the States." "I look forward to it, and enjoy your vacation," I communicate. After we hang up, I bow my head, thankful for having a friend that's a medical doctor who's willing to give me advice during this extremely challenging time in my life. I realize how truly blessed I am because I know not everyone in my position has a medical resource like Linda at their disposal.

Chapter 11
I Want the Robot

Excited to meet Dr. Sharp; I'm twenty minutes early for our March 23rd meeting. It's a good thing I am because I have to go to the restroom to empty my urine leg bag since it has gotten full and looks like it's about to burst. When I return, a nurse awaits me at the exam area's entrance. She takes me into the first room on the left near the nurses' station to check my vitals. Next, she uses a blood pressure cuff to check my pressure, a thermometer to read my temperature, and a stethoscope to listen to my breathing and heartbeat. When she's done, she tells me Dr. Sharp will see me soon.

Although I've never been operated on before, I'm not nervous about having prostate surgery. But I am anxious to get the surgery done and want my prostate out ASAP because I'm fearful the cancer is spreading! It's been highly frustrating these past four months because of COVID, everything in the healthcare sector; it seems, is taking forever to get things done. For example, it took Dr. Aminu nearly three weeks to schedule my first MRI because of a lack of equipment availability. I realize COVID patients are a priority and that hospitals are short-staffed and overworked right now, and I know it's selfish, but since I have cancer, I want to be tended to immediately! If my cancer starts

spreading rapidly and I die because of COVID delays, I'll be

cussing so much on my way to heaven that I might get sent

back down to the other place!

While waiting for Dr. Sharp, I check my cell phone for

email and text messages. A few minutes later, there's a knock

on the exam room's door. When I say, "Come in," in walks

two men. Dr. Sharp, who's not as tall as I had envisioned,

introduces himself first. Next, he introduces the other man,

who says, " Hello, " and tells me he's a resident medical

student. I wish the doctor-in-waiting well in his residency

and add, "From what I understand, you're being trained by

the best." Behind his mask, Dr. Sharp seems unimpressed

with my compliment, so I cease with the butt kissing. After

our introductions, Dr. Sharp asks me to tell him and the

resident something about myself. So I do, and as I'm

wrapping up, I tell them that Pooh and K.J. are both in the

medical field and enjoy what they are doing. "That's great,"

the two say.

"Before we review your treatment plan options, I'd like

to give you a rectal exam," Dr. Sharp says. Reluctantly, I say,

"Okay." After I pull down my pants and underwear, my first

thought is, 'I've had so many fingers and probes up my ass

these past few months; one more won't matter much.' With

his finger in my rectum, I can feel Dr. Sharp pressing my

prostate in different areas. He goes, "Un huh, okay, hmm, as I thought." He continues probing for what may have been less than a minute, but it feels like it's been an eternity. I'm relieved when he finishes, but as I pull up my underwear, Dr. Sharp tells me he'd also like the resident to perform a rectal examination. 'You've got to be kidding me,' I'm thinking. 'Two back-to-back rectal exams?'

So, grudgingly, I pull my shorts back down, lean over on the exam table, and as the future doctor moves his finger inside me, I have a sneaking suspicion that this is the first time he's done a rectal exam. To say he's a bit rough would be an understatement. The rookie's making my last exam with Dr. Aminu feel like a walk in the park. When I think things can't get any worse, Dr. Sharp instructs his mentee to examine the left side of my prostate further. I rise off the examination table as he does and say, "Ooh!" Then, the mentor tells his protege to examine my prostate's right side again. He does, and when the neophyte presses my prostate inward, I rise off the table again. Then, Dr. Sharp asks the newbie, "Now, do you see what I was talking about earlier?" The kid must not have understood because he says, "Hmm. Let me take a look at the left side again." 'Oh, no. Please, not again,' I'm thinking. As the youngster probes and presses my prostate, he's taking forever. Finally, to my immense relief, he says, "Yes, now I see what you mean." 'Thank

God,' I say to myself! The resident removes his finger, and the checkup is mercifully over.

After my two-for-one rectal exam, my butt's sore, so it takes me a moment to sit down. After I do, Dr. Sharp pulls up a chair, catty-corner to me, and gets seated. Next, he hands me a sheet of paper with multi-colored pictures. In the middle are four prostate images with numbers underneath that show T1-T4. On the immediate left, there's a box with the words, Your Tumor Stage = T2. As best as I can understand what he's telling me, this designation means my cancer is primarily confined to my prostate. On the top left of the page are two boxes with "Gleason Grading System Diagram" written at the top. And on the left, inside a rectangle, are the words, "Your Gleason Score (primary + secondary) = 8." When I ask what the number means, Dr. Sharp explains, and while I still don't quite understand, I know it's not good. So a lump builds up in my throat, and I'm getting extremely nervous. I have some questions for him, but I don't interrupt him further. Underneath the prostate photos are three rectangles with rounded corners. They stand out on the page because of their respective colors. The blue rectangle has a heading of Low, the green one, Intermediate, and the red, High. Underneath each title are the wording Tumor stage, Gleason sum, and PSA range. To his credit, Dr. Sharp notices that I'm confused, so he slows down for me. He points to the red rectangle where it shows "High Risk" and says, "That means some cancer has grown outside your prostate."

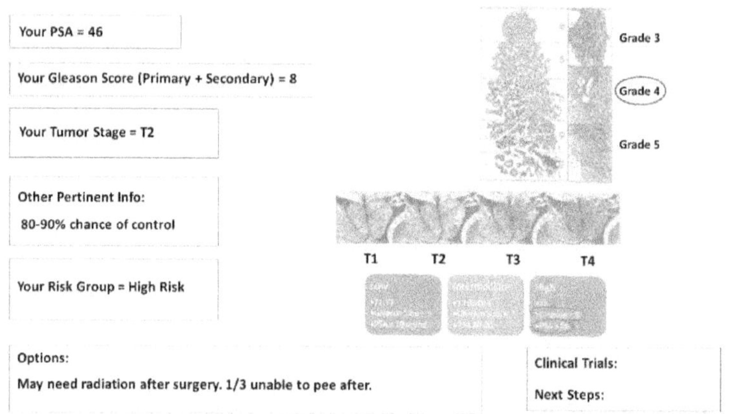

Data associated with the stage of my cancer

After Dr. Sharp finishes reviewing the sheet of paper with me, he lays out my treatment options which mirror what Dr. Aminu had told me earlier: surveillance, prostatectomy, or various forms of radiotherapy. He recommends a prostatectomy, which I agree with, so I tell him, "That's what I want to have done." Following, he says, "I'll arrange for the surgery." My heart is pounding, and my hands are sweating as I prepare to ask him the million-dollar question that's been on my mind these past four months. I clear my throat and nervously proceed by saying, "I won't hold you to this, but how much longer do I have to live after the surgery?" I'm nervously shaking the paper he gave me as I await his answer. After a pause, he finally says, "If any cancer remains after the surgery, you'll probably need to undergo 37 radiation treatments. However, if all goes well, data suggests there's an 80-90% chance your cancer can be controlled so that it doesn't shorten your life, excluding other things that may be unforeseen, of course."

The news that there's an 80-90% chance my cancer can be managed and not impact my life expectancy leaves me immediately overcome with joy and immense relief! It's as if the heavy burden I'd been bearing regarding my health status these past four months has been instantly lifted from my shoulders. Next, I lean forward and breathe a deep sigh of relief. Then I say, "That's the best news I've heard in months! Those are the words I wanted to hear!" "Well, I'm glad," Dr. Sharp says before he and the resident head for another appointment.

On my way home, I'm having difficulty driving because I'm constantly wiping tears of joy from my eyes. I thank God for today's news from Dr. Sharp because all I've wanted since my prognosis was a chance to live, and removing my cancerous prostate will give me that opportunity. We have a long embrace when I get home and tell Bay the news. After that, with tears in both of our eyes, I say, "My bright light is at work," and she says, "Yes, it is!" A few days later, I received a MyChart appointment notification showing Dr. Sharp had scheduled my prostate surgery for April 12th.

As I'm sitting in the lobby of Dr. Aminu's office two weeks later, waiting to attempt another void trial, boosted by Dr. Sharp's news, I've decided to tell the attending nurse I'll try self-catheterization again. So, when a nurse comes to get me, and while we're walking to an exam room, I say, "I'd like to skip the void trial today and try self-catheterizing at home. Before, I was afraid to try it, but now I'm convinced I can do it because I'm ready to get my life back. I'm tired of wearing a urinary leg bag, emptying it all day, and having it leak in public. I want more freedom of movement, and being able to self-catheterize will give me that." "That's the spirit, Mr. Simmons," the nurse says. "I'm sure you'll be able to self-catheterize when you get home, but if not, come back here, and we'll insert another catheter." "Don't worry," I tell her, "I don't plan on returning. The next time you see me, it'll be for something else. It won't be for another void trial or catheter insertion!" Nodding, the nurse says, "I hear you, Mr. Simmons."

When I get home, I rush downstairs to get ready to self-catheterize. Once in the bathroom, I peel back the plastic covering protecting the lubricated catheter and pull it out. Next, I turn the catheter so its green guide arrow points straight at me. I take a deep breath and mentally say,

'Whatever you do, don't force it in. Take it slow and easy, and don't stop until you reach your sphincter muscle.' After my self-help pep talk, I place the catheter in the opening of the head of my penis and start inserting the device in a slow, easy motion. Dammit, the guide arrow has turned. So, I start over, and the same thing happens after three or four attempts. Finally, it occurs to me that I'm going too slow and stopping too much versus proceeding continuously during the insertion. So I pull out the used catheter and grab a new one.

This time, I'm determined not to stop as the catheter passes through my urethra. Each time I try, I have a little bit more success, but attempt after attempt, every time I reach my sphincter muscle, it won't cooperate. Finally, I conclude I'm so uptight mentally about sticking something up my penis; I'm causing my sphincter to tighten when I get near it with the catheter, so I'm going to take a thirty-minute break and try to relax.

After my break, I return to the bathroom, open the packaging of my third or fourth catheter, and restart my insertion attempt. It's been two and a half hours since I started, and I still have no luck. And, if things couldn't get worse, my bladder is full and feels like it's about to burst. I've spent so much time trying to self-catheterize; I've reached a point where I'm now in a potentially life-threatening situation, and I'm starting to fear my bladder might rupture. I'm up Shit's Creek and have to do something fast! I've got two choices. I can return to Dr. Aminu's office right now and let a nurse put a catheter in me, which means I'll have to continue wearing a leg bag to capture my urine. After my leaking incident at Kroger, there's no way I want to continue wearing one of those damn things. Or, I can give self-catheterization one or two more tries before heading back to Dr. Aminu's office or the emergency room. I'm going with option two. I have to make this work because time is running out, and if I fail, I'm in a world of hurt, so I've got to get this fricking pee device in me, even if it kills me!

So, for the umpteenth time, as I begin inserting a new catheter into the head of my penis, I'm focusing on the green triangle to ensure the catheter is inserted correctly and straight. I take a deep breath, and in a slow continuous inward motion, I keep moving the catheter up and inside my urethra. When it hits my sphincter muscle, I try to relax. But unfortunately, my sphincter muscle and I are still at a standstill. I'm knocking on its door, but it won't let me in. Now, my bladder is screaming! Convinced I'm in a do-or-I-may-die situation if my bladder bursts, I say aloud, "You've got to get this catheter into your bladder, and you got to do it right now!"

With the catheter touching my sphincter, I push with slightly more force, and when I do, it feels like I've pricked the muscle a little. When I look at the green triangle, dammit, the catheter has shifted slightly to the right. I quickly straighten it and press it against my sphincter muscle again, pushing more forcefully, and when I do, to my astonishment, the catheter makes it through my sphincter. I can't believe it! I've managed to get through the "shut door," and the catheter is inside my bladder! Right away, urine starts running through the catheter's clear plastic tubing. I breathe a huge sigh of relief. After numerous attempts, I've finally self-catheterized! A pee never felt so good! After emptying my bladder, I inhale deeply and quickly pull the catheter out. Taking it out is a hell of a lot easier than putting the SOB in! There's a little blood on the device's tip where I nicked the sphincter, but the slight nick was worth it. No more leg bags, hooray! When Bay gets home, I tell her about my success, and she's almost as happy as I am.

Following my self-catheterizing success, curious about how many others have to do it, I take it to Google. An article I find says, "The World Health Organization estimates that more than 200 million people have bladder control problems, with many needing to use urinary catheters." That's when reality hits me like a ton of bricks. What a whiner I've been these past few months. My catheter use will probably be short-term, at least I hope it is, and here I am complaining about having to use one. What about those paralyzed from the waist down or those who've lost their legs? Millions of people, I would imagine, have to utilize catheters for the rest of their lives, and here I am bitching and moaning. Suddenly, my appreciation for catheter users grows by leaps and bounds. From now on, I'm done with complaining about catheter use because my plight could be much worse.

Chapter 12
My Prostate Removal

A few days before my prostate surgery, I had a voicemail from an Emory Healthcare staffer who had called to give me my pre-surgery instructions. When I called her back, some instructions she gave me were to arrive at the hospital by 11:15 A.M. but no later than noon, not eat past midnight the day before the procedure, and bathe or shower with antibacterial soap. And after my hospital stay, I would need someone to drive me home. The night before my surgery, I could hardly sleep for wondering about the procedure's outcome. Would Dr. Sharp be able to get all of the cancer, or did some of it on the periphery of my prostate get out and spread?

On the morning of April 12th, I wake up at 6:00 A.M. feeling spry and optimistic about a positive outcome once my prostate is removed. Once in the shower with my gold bar Dial antibacterial soap, I wash and rinse myself four times, then once more for good measure because I want to be squeaky clean before my surgery. I plan on driving to the hospital, but Bay insists on chauffeuring me, so reluctantly, I give in to her request. While standing in the kitchen together, we hold hands, bow our heads and say a prayer before we head out.

Once in the car and before the garage door opens, I ask Bay again, "Are you sure you don't want me to drive? I-285 will be a zoo heading into the lunch hour," I tell her. "I'll be all right," she says. When we reach the I-285 W exit and head up the ramp, all six westbound lanes are bumper to bumper. I can tell Bay's nervous because she's holding both hands on the stirring wheel so tight that her knuckles turn red. So I say, "Try to relax. I'll keep looking back and let you know when you can merge into traffic." Shortly after that, an opening appears, and I say, "This guy is letting you in." So, she turns on her left turn single and slowly winds into the lane adjacent to our oncoming ramp. Once Bay is in the traffic flow, we wave at the car behind us, thanking the driver for letting us in. As I look ahead, traffic is backed up to the Peachtree Dunwoody Road exit. Looking at the map on my phone, Bay and I are in a three-mile parking lot! So now I'm thinking, 'We'll be at least thirty minutes late.' I'm not saying a word because I don't want to make Bay more nervous than she already is.

While we're sitting in traffic, Bay turns down the car radio and asks me if I'm nervous about the surgery, and I confide, "As strange as it may seem, I'm not. On the contrary, I'm comforted knowing I'm being "watched over" by the bright light I saw. But I wonder, "What if I can't urinate after the surgery? Will I have to be on a catheter for the rest of my life? I don't know if I'll be able to handle that." Then, reassuringly, Bay says, "Don't worry. I'm sure that you will be able to urinate, so claim it!" "Okay, I'm claiming it," I reply. "And when everything is all said and done, I will shout from the rooftops what God has done for me and share the miracle he's performed inside me with others."

When we finally arrive at the hospital, as we drive past its entrance and begin looking for parking, I forget to tell Bay we can park in the purple area for cancer patients. So we end up in the general parking lot, which is always filled, and today is no exception. So as Bay winds through the various rows, I tell her our best bet is to park in the lower level. Unfortunately, once there, it's jam-packed too. Finally, a car backs out, and Bay pulls into the vacated space.

After we get to the two sets of double glass doors at the hospital's entrance, a gust of wind follows us when the first set of doors opens, so a man wearing a hat has to grab it to keep it from flying off. When I look at him and say, "Our apologies," he nods; and says, "That's okay," as he tips his hat to us. Once we get through the second set of doors, there are two receptionists to our left. One is helping someone, and the other waves us over. I tell her I'm here for surgery, so she directs me to the check-in area to our right and across from the middle of the lobby. The lobby's pretty crowded, so

Bay and I look for seating first. Once we find two seats, I put my backpack in one, and Bay sits in the other.

When I walk up to the check-in line, there's one person ahead of me. Less than a minute later, I get waved up by a receptionist. She asks me for my date of birth and time of surgery. After I give her the information, a wristband prints out on a small blue printer next to her computer keyboard. She hands me the bracelet and asks me to check it for accuracy, so I look at the white plastic wristlet and acknowledge that my name and date of birth are correct. After that, she puts the bracelet on my wrist. I hate these things because the edges are sharp, and I always forget to take the bracelet off and end up showcasing it in public, which I find embarrassing. The hospital bracelets also get placed too close to my wrist, so I always have difficulty getting scissors underneath them to cut them off. But, as inconvenient as they are, I can see the benefit because I sure as hell wouldn't want to be taken into brain or heart surgery today by mistake!

Before I head back to my seat, the receptionist says, "Mr. Simmons, if you would like something to drink, there's a café behind you straight down the hall. Remember, though, you can't have anything to eat before your surgery." So, I returned to my seat and asked Bay if she would like anything from the café, and she said, "No, thank you, I'm fine." Her eyebrows raise when I tell her I'm going to grab some coffee because she knows I rarely ever drink coffee. It's so cold in the lobby from the front doors opening and closing, though; I need something to warm me up, I tell her. As I'm finishing my coffee, a nurse walks out from behind the reception area, calls my name, and I say, "Here!" I look at Bay and tell her my procedure could take hours and that there's no need for her to sit for who knows how long waiting on me. "Why don't you head home? I'll have a nurse call you after my surgery, and I've been put in a room," I verbalize. She asks, "Are you sure? Are you going to be all right?" When I tell her I'll be fine, we hug and kiss one another goodbye.

As the nurse and I head through some double doors, I ask God to guide Dr. Sharp's hands and that I have a safe surgery. Following, the nurse takes me into a small examination room with a gurney, tv, and some medical devices. After I put my backpack in a chair, she asks me to remove my clothes, then hands me a hospital gown and some socks to keep my feet warm. When I'm done, she checks my vitals. Afterward, as she's typing my readings into a computer, there's a knock on the door, so we both say, "Come in."

Another nurse and an anesthesiologist enter the exam room and introduce themselves. After that, the anesthesiologist reviews my chart to confirm the medications I'm currently taking. Once verified, he tells me the anesthetic he'll be using will be administered intravenously and that I'll drift off to sleep shortly. "You can go ahead and start Mr. Simmons' IV drip," he tells the original nurse. Then, he asks me if I have any questions, and I tell him I don't. Next, as he's shaking my hand on his way out, he says, "I'll see you in the operating room." Shortly after that, everything goes dark.

My eyelids open slowly, and I hear rolling wheels. I can feel myself bouncing on something. When I look up, I see ceiling tile and realize I'm being rolled down a hall on a gurney. Looking to my left, I see the two nurses who told me they'd assist Dr. Sharp in the operating room, moving me along. "Thank you. You guys and Dr. Sharp just saved my life," I mumble. "How did everything go? Where are you taking me?" They both answer, "You did great!" Then one says, "We're taking you to your room now."

When we got to my room, one of the nurses had to leave for another surgery, so the remaining nurse asked if she could get me anything. "I'm thirsty and would like some water," I say. When she asks me if I'd like a little or a lot of ice, I reply, "Just a little, please." When the nurse returns, she tells me Dr. Sharp will be in to see me shortly. Later, while a phlebotomist takes a blood sample from me, there's a knock on the door. When I say, "Come in," in walks Dr. Sharp.

"Hi, Mr. Simmons. How do you feel?"

"Thank you for saving my life. I feel fine, but my abdomen is sore."

"That's to be expected. I used six small incisions to remove your prostate. I'll have the nurse get you something for the pain. Well, you're probably wondering how things went with your surgery."

"Yes, I am."

"Well, yours was a complex procedure that took several hours to complete and was much more complex than usual, but you did fine."

"Do you think I'll be able to urinate now?"

"We'll know in a few weeks. Although I like your chances, there's no guarantee. And as I shared with you earlier, we have some options for you if you can't."

"Are you talking about the button that can be placed on my abdomen that I can push to pee?"

"Yes, that's one of the options, but let's see how you do over the next few weeks. Get some rest, and I'll have my staff schedule another appointment for you in a week."

After Dr. Sharp leaves, my first thought is, 'Damn, he's good!' Later, when dinner time comes, I order my meal from the cafeteria and request a key lime pie for dessert. Bay, Pooh, and K.J. visited me shortly after I finished my dinner. I told them Dr. Sharp had stopped by and that things went well with my surgery. The three are very pleased with the news.

Bay asks me if I've eaten dinner, and I tell her I have and that I also had key lime pie for dessert. Following, out of nowhere, Pooh bursts out laughing, saying, "Lord Dad, you know you love yourself some key lime pie." She's referring to my previous nine-day hospital stay, where I had key lime pie for lunch and dinner every day for over a week. I had told Pooh I had eaten so much of the dessert that one day when I placed my order, the cafeteria's dietician chastised me and said, "Mr. Simmons. You're eating way too much key lime pie. I can't let you have any more. You can have a fruit popsicle, but no more key lime pie!" During their stay, I thank Bay, Pooh, and K.J. for their love and support these past five months. I tell them that without theirs and the prayers of others, I probably wouldn't be here today. Then, we all shed some tears, and each comes to my bed and hugs me.

The following morning, after I've eaten breakfast, Dr. Sharp drops by to check in on me. First, he updates me on my vitals and shares that they look fine for the most part. Next, he tells me that his robotic prostatectomy patients are typically released after twenty-four hours of observation. But my vitals indicate I'm a little hypoglycemic, so he wants to prescribe something to increase my blood sugar level. As a result, I'll need to stay in the hospital another night, and if my level improves, he expects he'll probably release me tomorrow around noon. After he leaves, I call Bay with an update so she can be on standby to pick me up.

Chapter 13
My Right Shoulder Angel Returns

Late mid-afternoon, a phlebotomist wanting to take some blood wakes me from my nap. I'm convinced there's been a camera in every one of my Emory Healthcare hospital rooms with an alarm that flags someone to come in and wake me up so I can't go to sleep! So, half awake, I let the tech get his blood, and when he leaves, I lie back down to resume my nap. I don't know how long I've been asleep, but suddenly I feel the bed shake and am awakened by something. Then, out of nowhere - an enormous tan wing appears before my eyes. I'm sure I'm not hallucinating because it has been over twenty-four hours since I was anesthetized. When I try lifting my right arm a little, I can't move it or my other arm or legs, but I can move my head. Looking at the wing, I think, 'People won't believe me when I tell them about this.' And, as happened in the emergency room, I know I'm lucid and coherent. I also realize I'm now undergoing my second "divine" experience. And just as I did when the bright light appeared in the emergency room, I tell myself, 'You've got to concentrate on everything happening and mentally record it.' Looking at the wing, I'm convinced it's my right shoulder angel, and she's returned. But I can't figure out why she's presenting herself to me so pronounced. I mean, this wing is enormous! Previously, the angel was smaller than an elf when she lightly floated on my right shoulder. Next, the wing moves slowly and closer toward the head of my bed. I'm becoming frightened because I know I'll suffocate if it plops down on me. Then, it stops moving and is still.

I'm looking at the underside of the wing, and all but a few feathers are tan. The non-tan ones are brown. Next, I shift my focus to the front of the appendage nearest my eyes. It looks like thick cartilage with smooth tan feathers layering it. Now the wing moves slowly toward the head of my bed again. Soon my head and torso are entirely underneath it. It's about four inches above my eyes. I can tell it's the angel's right wing, not the left, because its width is narrower at the end as I look toward my left. Plus, if it were the left wing, I'd be able to see the end of the appendage and the wall on my right, but I can't see either.

Instantly, I think, 'First, God came into my emergency room area and shone a bright light. Now, I'm looking at this massive angel's wing.' The first "sign" I received had to have been an affirmation of God's presence. The angel's wing must be a reaffirmation. Now I'm more convinced than ever that I'm not about to die soon. God is saving me for a reason. But I don't know what it is. During both "sightings," my first thought was to capture everything mentally, 'So, am I supposed to write about my two experiences? Or am I supposed to "spread the gospel" about my upcoming "healing?" What is it that I'm supposed to do with these two "divine signs" I've received? I don't know what God wants me to do, but I'm sure he's saving me for some purpose. I don't know what it is yet.' After my brief wondering, the angel's wing slowly lifts and disappears, and when it does, I can move my arms and legs again.

After the angel's wing departed, I thought, 'My right shoulder angel is tiny, but this one was large and felt like a different angel. I wonder if it was my mom. Did she come back to tell me I would be okay?' Immediately after my angel's wing experience, I wrote down what I had witnessed in a composition book that I use for writing down notes and reminders when I'm conducting business and that Bay had brought me from home. In it, I wrote, "Surgery went well. Saw a large wing that was tan and brown but mostly tan. I was lucid and had talked to a nurse just before I had fallen to sleep." After that, I wondered, 'If I was hallucinating, would I be able to write a note about my experience right after the event?' I don't think I would.

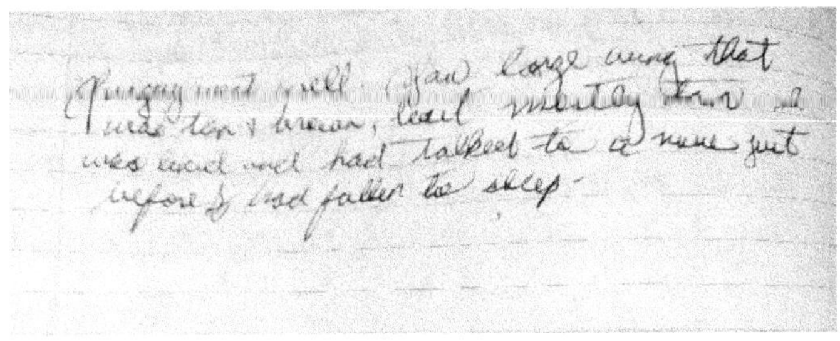

Photo of my angel's wing notes taken from my hospital bed.

After encountering the angel's wing, an inner peace overwhelms me almost immediately. This feeling is unlike any I've ever experienced before. It's as if my inner body has been cleansed. I feel like I'm in a weightless chamber, floating on air without a care. Realizing I've now had two "reassurances" that I won't die from my cancer, I've got to make the most of my life. And with my second chance at life, I know I better not screw this one up! So, the first thing I must do is to listen to my doctors, do what they say and get well.

Night comes, and when Bay stops by to visit me, we kiss, and afterward, she asks me how my day went. When I tell her about the angel's wing I saw, she says, "That's God at work, Eric," and I reply, "Yes, He is!" When my dinner arrives, and as I'm talking to Bay, I look over at the chair she's sitting in, and she's fallen sound asleep. Between me, and her sister's passing, she's exhausted. Man, I've got to get well soon. My situation is draining Bay. So, I let her sleep for a while, but when it gets late, I wake her up, saying, "Why don't you go home and get some rest? I'll be fine. Plus, I believe Dr. Sharp's releasing me in the morning, so we'll have plenty of time to spend together when I get home." Yawning with both arms outstretched, she slowly rises from her chair and says, "Okay, call me tomorrow and let me know when they're releasing you." I assure her I will.

After Bay leaves and I'm all alone, I figure it's time for my cancer and I to chat. So, I close my eyes and concentrate on the inside of my body. It's quiet there, and I mostly see dark brownish-orange colors. Next, I mentally start saying to my cancer, 'I don't know if you're still in me, but I will beat you. Hear me and hear now cancer. I am going to whip you! A bright light and the right wing of an angel already have made it so!'

The next day, as I'm watching the morning news, I'm getting depressed by what I'm seeing, so I turn the tv off. Then, alone with my thoughts, I ask myself, 'If someone were to ask me what's it been like these past five months, what would I tell them?' As I contemplate my question, I envision a sports analogy I might tell people.

"My journey with prostate cancer has been like playing tug-of-war on a sandy beach. On one side, you have the devil and my prostate cancer. Me, the bright light I saw, and the right angel's wing are on the other side. In between both teams, there is a white line. So, the game's object, using a large, coarse brown rope, similar to a mooring line used to dock a boat but much thicker, is to pull the other team over the white line. Once done, you win but lose if pulled over the line.

But this isn't your regular tug-of-war, and it isn't a mere game. Instead, this is a high-stakes contest that's played for keeps! So, If my team and I get pulled across the line, I'll probably lose my faith, end up with my cancer progressing, and die. So as the game progresses, despite seemingly being outnumbered with only two players, my prostate cancer and the devil are powerful. Before the referee blows his whistle to start the match, the devil and my prostate cancer pull on the rope, surprising my team and me! Now we're straining and agonizing as we hold onto the rope to keep me from getting pulled over the line. Then, we pull hard, wincing in pain as we walk backward with the rope. Now the devil and prostate cancer begin sliding toward us and the white marker. The teams see-saw back and forth, losing and gaining ground. My hands have developed rope burns, and my feet are blistering from being dragged across the sand. And when I'm exhausted and want to quit, the bright light and the angel's wing prop me back up."

Yep! Something along those lines is what I might tell people about my prostate cancer experience.

While I'm eating lunch, there's a knock on the door. I say, "Come in," and Doctor Sharp enters my room. He tells me my blood sugar level has dropped to a desirable level and that he's made arrangements for my release at 2:00 P.M. today. After I thank him again for "saving my life," as, what appears to be his demeanor, he shies away from receiving credit for the positive impact he's had on my life. However, since he's alluded to my situation being complex on two occasions, I sense mine was one of the most, if not the most, challenging prostatectomies he's ever performed. As a result, I think he's immensely proud he was up to the challenge and achieved a successful operation on me. Before he heads out, when I tell him I hope the surgery got all the prostate cancer, he replies, "We won't know until your PSA results return." Then, as we bid one another goodbye, he says, "I'll see you in a few weeks." After Dr. Sharp departs, I loudly exhale, "Whew!" I'm relieved the surgery is over, and I can go home. I can finally call Bay to let her know she can pick me up.

When Bay arrived, she helped me finish gathering my things. As we were doing so, the attending nurse entered the room and said she would get me a wheelchair, so Bay left to get the car. I didn't realize how sore my midsection was until I had to get up from the wheelchair and sit down in the car when Bay pulled it up in front of the hospital. After we leave the hospital, thankfully, there's no rush hour traffic on our way home, so, traffic-wise, the drive is uneventful.

I'm so physically and mentally exhausted from the surgery and the stressful five months I've been through that I head straight to bed once we're home. Around 6:00 P.M. or so, Bay wakes me up to eat. She's brought me dinner on a tray, so I wouldn't have to walk up and down the stairs from the basement. When I tell her my post-surgery information sheet recommends that I do light walking to build my strength back up, she says, "Well, you can start after you eat." Determined to help me improve, Bay waits on me hand over fist for the next few weeks. She's preparing huge salads and ensuring I eat three square meals daily. Resolved to regain weight, I'm supplementing my diet with vanilla organic protein shake powder and Ensure. To help my kidneys improve, I'm drinking seventy-two ounces of water daily, as my nephrologist prescribes. Now that my stomach is no longer "scrunched up," I have an appetite again, and I'm eating like a horse! And as my dissolvable stitches from surgery disappear one by one, I feel better by the day. Finally, after two weeks, all my stitches dissolved, and I'm no longer sore in my pelvic area from my surgery. Admittedly, I'm stunned that my recovery is going so well.

I'm getting anxious as May 4th nears because that's the day I'll learn if my prostate removal surgery was successful to the extent that I'll be able to pee without a catheter. The upcoming void trial will be another "moment of truth," as being told I had prostate cancer, my nuclear bone scan, getting my 3D MRI scan, and biopsy results have been others. My upcoming ability or inability to urinate is another "do or die" situation, in my opinion. 'What if I can't urinate? What comes next? Will I have to use a catheter for the rest of my life? If not, and I elect to have a mechanical "button" placed in my abdomen to urinate, is it going to be awkward operating it if I'm over to someone's house and I need to use the bathroom to pee?' These and other questions are flooding my mind. While I'm doing my best to stay positive and trust in the bright light and right angel wing, my previous void trials have been such a disaster that I can't bear the thought of another failed attempt.

Bay takes a day off to be with me for my void trial. She can tell I'm nervous, so while encouraging me, my left shoulder angel is hard at work. He's telling me I won't be able to pee, and I believe him. He's humming in my ear and repeating, "Nanna, nanna booboo, Butch will have to wear a catheter for the rest of his life." Because I don't hear a peep from my right shoulder angel, I say to Bay, "I doubt I'll be able to urinate today. I don't think I will be able to do it."

"Nonsense," she replies. "The God I know says you will. You've come too far, so you can't give up now." Finally, to appease her, I say, "You're right. I've got to believe I'll pee on my own today." These are shallow words, though, because I'm highly unoptimistic.

When we arrived at the hospital, I remember to let Bay know we could park in the purple lot for cancer patients. After we park and I check-in, we take the elevator upstairs to the first floor, where the Department of Urology is located. After a short wait, a nurse named Monica comes to get me. After I introduced her to Bay, Monica took us down a hall and into an exam room on the left. I told her I wouldn't forget her name because I have a niece with the same name. After Monica reviews my medical information and checks my bracelet to ensure I'm the correct patient, she begins conversing with Bay and me. The three of us hit off right away. After voicing my concern that I won't be able to pee, Monica says, "Don't worry, Mr. Simmons. After their surgery, I've seen patients urinate on the first try. For some, it takes two or three attempts. Unfortunately, some can't urinate, but something tells me you'll pee on your first try." Monica's encouraging words are helpful, but I'm still pessimistic. Next, she hands me a hospital gown and says, "Now take off your shoes, pants, and underwear and lie on your back on the exam table, please." I'm as nervous as hell when I sit on the table and put my left leg on it to prepare to lie down.

As I'm lying on my back, my mind wanders. I'm thinking about the hell I've been through these past six months and that Death has looked me right in the eye and hasn't blinked. I recall the countless sleepless nights I've had because of those hard-assed plastic nephrostomy tubes hanging down my back and my back constantly itching. Both scenarios caused me to have suicidal thoughts on several occasions. And I can still hear the biopsy "staple gun's" clicking sound. Man, I wouldn't want anyone to go through what I've gone through these past six months. So, now everything has boiled down to this moment. Will I or won't I be able to pee following my prostate surgery?

As nurse Monica connects a twelve-ounce bottle of saline solution to my catheter, she tells me she'll be emptying the entire bottle into my bladder. So, as the bottle drains, I tell her I can feel my bladder getting full. Then, unexpectedly and without forewarning, she abruptly says, "Yes, Mr. Simmons, I believe you're going to urinate on your first try. There, the catheter's out!" "You're kidding! I didn't feel a thing," I tell her. I've had several catheter changes, and I could always feel it when my catheter was removed. But this time, I didn't feel anything! "Boy, you're good," I express to her.

Next, Monica says, "Okay, Mr. Simmons, I'm going to give you a urine jug, and I want you to place the opening over your penis, then slowly sit up for me and try to pee." So, when I start sitting up, some clear urine trickles into the jug. Immediately I attribute the small amount of urine to leftover saline from the catheter's removal. Then, as I turn to position myself on the bed's edge, there are more pee trickles. Next, when I stand up, incredibly urine begins to flow! I can't believe my eyes! "The surgery worked," I say to Bay and Monica. "Thank you, Lord. Thank you." Now, I'm crying a river of tears, and after emptying my bladder, Bay runs across the room and bear-hugs me. We're both crying tears of joy. I'm so proud of my accomplishment that I ask Bay to please hand me my camera so I can take a picture of my urine in the jug for keepsake. After taking my photo, I notice Monica standing by the door, so I motion her to join us in a group hug. Now, she's crying too.

On our drive home, I tell Bay, "It feels like an enormous boulder has been taken off my shoulders." Once at home, I'm so emotionally drained that I head straight to bed to "decompress." But, once in bed, I can't help but think about how we take something so routine as peeing for granted. After all that I've been through, I doubt I'll take peeing for granted again! Now that I no longer have to rely on a catheter to help me urinate, I face another new challenge.

Having worn a catheter for six months, I haven't been using my pelvic muscles, which, combined with my prostate surgery, has left me unable to control my bladder. So now, I will have to wear what the hospital staff calls incontinence underwear, which, in my opinion, is just a glorified name for fitted diapers. I know I shouldn't be complaining because at least I'm peeing again, but I'm wondering, 'How long will I have to wear these "diapers?" Is my incontinence going to be short or long-term?' I hope it's short-term because I'm going through five or six incontinence underwear daily. And they're hot, expensive, and not covered by our insurance. But then again, changing my "diapers" beats self-catheterizing any day!

Chapter 14
The Cancer Has Spread

Before my prostate surgery, my PSA level had peaked at 46.59 ng/ml, which is incredibly high (i.e., over nine (9) times higher than the average for a Black man my age, per the National Library of Medicine)! However, after my surgery, and on my birthday, May 19th, my post-surgery blood work came back, and my PSA had dropped to 0.61, which is well within the 0-5.5 ng/ml range that's considered normal for my age group, per the previously referenced source. Talk about a great birthday gift! And although Dr. Sharp wants my PSA level to be at 0.00, I'm ecstatic that most of my cancer appears to be gone and that only a little bit is left.

Unfortunately, a month later, my PSA level has risen to 0.65 ng/ml and 0.73 several months after. 'Oh, shit,' I think! I don't need Dr. Sharp or Dr. Aminu to tell me this isn't good because I know the number should not be increasing; it should be decreasing! 'So, did some cancer that showed up in previous imaging on the outer membrane of my prostate get out? If so, how much? Is it spreading, and if it is, to what extent?' The thought of some cancer "leaking" out and that it could be spreading demoralizes me. The emotional strain of "tug-of-war" is back on, and I don't know how much more of this seemingly unending psychological rollercoaster ride I can take. I'm at my wit's end now, and if I had any hair, I'd pull it out!

As I'm trying to calm myself down by listening to my YouTube playlist, as if ordained, an ad for St. Jude's Children's Hospital comes on. When a picture of a bald child comes up and fades to his mother, who's talking about how unfair it is for a child to have cancer, I'm brought to tears. Suddenly, I'm ashamed of my lack of courage and constant complaining about my situation when this child exhibits far more courage than I do! If there's anyone who doesn't deserve cancer, it's a child. As I watch the video, I can't imagine what his parents must be going through. But, inspired by the child's bravery, I tell myself, 'You've got to persevere. You've got a bright light and an angel's right wing watching over you, so you've got to try and live, if not for yourself, but for the kids and Bay because Lord knows she'd be heartbroken without you.'

With my PSA level increasing, Dr. Sharp has scheduled a meeting with me on August 17th, the day before Bay's and my wedding anniversary, to revisit my treatment plan. During our meeting, he introduces me to Dr. Denton, a radiation oncologist, with whom I hit it off immediately. The two recommend I have another Nuclear whole-body bone scan to see if the cancer cells have invaded my bones. 'Here we go again,' I say to myself. Afterward, I would have a

PSMA PET scan, a more precise method to determine the location of my cancerous prostate cells. "And, if the cells are still localized in your pelvic region, you will undergo a month of hormone treatment followed by five days a week of radiation treatment for seven weeks," Dr. Denton says. But, since prostate cancer thrives on testosterone, he tells me another treatment method would be to "starve" the cancerous cells by lowering my testosterone level. After that, Dr. Sharp asked me if I would be interested in a clinical trial study, provided he could get me into it. It would involve me taking a testosterone-reducing pill during my hormone therapy versus a Lupron injection, the more common treatment method for lowering a patient's testosterone. I'm somewhat familiar with Lupron because Bay's Uncle took injections for his prostate cancer. Unfortunately, one of the side effects he experienced was hot flashes, which is, apparently, typical for the drug. I didn't want to go through the same, so I elected to participate in the clinical trial.

When I got home, I was devastated about having another bone scan. 'If cancer has spread to my bones - I've just been served a death sentence,' I think! The emotional back and forth I'm going through has been going on for so long now; more and more, it's taking a mental and physical toll on me. It's wearing me down and testing my patience to the core.

Days before my second Nuclear bone scan, scheduled for August 29th, I'm nervous "as hell" and much more so than before my first Nuclear scan. Ultimately, on the day of my scan, I'm void of feelings as I'm lying in the chamber of the scanner. I'm beginning to lose my fight and will to live. I can't imagine death being much worse than I've been going through. But then I realized it boils down to allowing my doctors to take all these medical precautions and do all of this testing, or I could die. I ask myself, 'But what about kids with cancer? What about Bay and our children?' Then I think, 'I need to stop feeling sorry for myself, and I've got to fight this thing even if it does kill me. I've got to stick around long enough to share God's grace and mercy toward me with others. I've got to let them know about how He healed me. So, before I get all worked up about cancer possibly being in my bones, I need to pray it isn't.' And so I do, and the scan is over soon after that.

When I get home, I'm so anxious to see the results from my bone scan; I check MyChart every few hours, and each time nothing's there. Waiting for significant test results, like a bone scan, is about as excruciating for me as the nephrostomy tubes were when they were hanging from my back. And like with the plastic cylinders, I keep asking myself, "Will my plight ever end? When will all of this be over?" It has been several days now, and I can't figure out why the bone scan results are taking so long. I sure hope they haven't found cancer in my bones. Finally, a few days later, as I review the "Test Results" section in MyChart, a line item reads, "NM Bone Scan Whole Body."

At last, the results of my bone scan are back! My heart's pounding, and a lump develops in my throat, so before reviewing the scan results, I pray, 'Lord, please don't let cancer be in my bones.' Then I nervously click on the link to see the bone scan findings. Once I'm on the page containing the results, there's a good bit of medical jargon that I don't understand. But when I see the wording, "…there are no discrete foci of abnormal radiotracer uptake highly concerning for osseous metastatic disease," I somewhat understand what it means. Recalling my old anatomy classes, osseous has something to do with bones and likewise metastatic with cancer. Next, I have to Google the meaning of foci, and when I do, I learn it means the center of interest or activity. So, when I piece everything together, I'm pretty sure the information says the test results came back "negative," Thank God! After that, I let out a prolonged "Whew," collapse in my office chair, and start crying, so it takes me about ten minutes to collect myself before texting Bay and the kids with the update. Of course, Bay is the first to reply. "That's excellent news," she writes! Then, over the next thirty minutes, all three kids respond with a similar message. So now, I have one crucial hurdle down and one to go: my PSMA Pet Scan. A few days following my bone scan, I receive a MyChart email stating I have a new appointment. So, when I log in, my calendar shows I have a PSMA PET Scan appointment on September 21st.

Three weeks later, on the day of my PSMA PET Scan, when I got to the hospital, a nurse led me through the facility and out into the rear parking lot where a sizeable mobile trailer sat about twenty feet from the door we exited. I'm thinking, 'What the hay?' So I ask, "Why's the scanner out here?" The nurse says, "It was moved to accommodate COVID patients." "That makes sense," I reply. After we entered the trailer, the nurse handed me off to another nurse who told me she would be responsible for taking my images today.

Next, the "scanning" nurse takes me to the right side of the trailer, where a partition separates two oversized green recliners. The recliner in front of us is occupied by another patient up next for a scan. So, the nurse directed me to the other chair on our left. Once settled in my chair, the nurse hands me a white twenty-ounce Styrofoam cup filled with ice and a liquid. She tells me that after I drink the whole cup, I'll have to wait thirty minutes before she can do the scan. I start sipping on the drink, which tastes like Gatorade but chalky. As I'm sipping the concoction, I start conversing with the nurse as she's putting some medicine in a cabinet.

"Am I drinking a radioactive isotope to cause my prostate cancer to light up when the images are taken?"

"Yes. How did you know that?"

"I used to sell diagnostic imaging equipment for GE's Medical Systems unit, but I never sold PET scanners. So it seems logical that the fluid I'm drinking will cause my cancerous cells to light up or "glow" while the scanner takes images."

"That's about right. Well, if you don't need anything now, I'm heading to my desk to start the other patient's scan, and I'll return in about thirty minutes to prepare you for your scan. But don't hesitate to come get me if you need me."

"Okay, I don't need anything right now, and I'll do my best to try not to disturb you."

About twenty minutes later, the nurse came to get me for my scan. I asked her, "Wasn't it supposed to be thirty minutes before I was scanned?" She says enough time has passed for the fluid to be in my system. Afterward, she takes me to the scanner and has me lie on the patient's table. Once on the table, she asks me to stretch my arms out backward, like Superman would look if he were flying upside down. Next, she asks me if I need anything else before she starts, and I tell her I don't. Then, as the table slowly moves me toward the scanner's opening, my thought is, 'If the unit is as precise as Dr. Sharp mentioned, we'll know from the "hot spots" on the images if my cancer has spread to other non-bone parts of my body.'

After about fifteen minutes inside the scanner, both my arms start aching where they connect to my shoulders. I have to concentrate hard now on not moving because if I do, I'll distort the images, and goodness knows; I don't want to come back for another scan. Suddenly, the scanner stops, and the nurse asks me to turn over halfway on my right side so I'm perpendicular to the table. After I do, she pivots the scanner semi-circle to take more images. So, instead of the unit being one round piece of equipment, as it appears, it's two half pieces, which I think is pretty cool. When she finishes scanning me, she has me turn halfway on my left side, then resumes scanning using the scanner's other half to take images.

A few days later, my PSMA PET Scan results are posted on MyChart. And once again, I don't understand all of the medical terminology. But from what I can glean, something has shone up around two ribs and behind my bladder. I broke a rib playing football in elementary school during recess, so I think that's probably one of the "hot spots" that's showing. Hopefully, the other spot on the other rib is just an anomaly, and any remaining cancerous cells are still localized in my pelvic region. When I tell Bay and Pooh how difficult the chart notes are to read, Dr. Pooh, as I sometimes call her, says, "Dad, to better understand the imaging results, review the "Impression" section." So, I go back downstairs, open the "View Notes" section, and look for the "Impression" segment. Once there, the information reveals the "hot spots" on my ribs are cancerous cells, and they've also spread to the right side of my T4 vertebrae, midway up my spine. I'm devastated!

Later, during a meeting with Dr. Denton on September 28th, he confirmed my understanding of the "Impression" information I had read in MyChart. My cancer had indeed spread, and cancerous cells were present on my seventh left rib, which I thought might be an anomaly, on my right sixth rib, behind my bladder, and in my T4 vertebrae. As a result, he says, my treatment plan must be changed. Upon hearing the news, I'm overcome with sadness and fear. I strain as tears well up in my eyes to keep them from streaming down my face. Now more than ever, I'm sure I'll have to undergo chemotherapy, which I'm deathly afraid of going through. Finally, tears start trickling down my cheeks, so I wipe them off, clear my throat, and ask Dr. Denton if I must undergo chemo. Without hesitating, he says, "No!" After that, I breathe a deep sigh of relief and say, "Whew!"

Next, he tells me I have what is referred to as "advanced" prostate cancer, but that mine is treatable with radiation. However, rather than start radiation treatment immediately, he suggests I undergo hormone therapy for two to three months to see if that will kill the cancerous cells. After that, he plans to consult with his colleagues to see if radiation treatment is necessary. So, for the time being, he will be referring me to Dr. Hoffman, an oncologist he respects immensely and highly recommends for my hormone treatment. After he finished, relieved, I told him, "I'm so glad I won't have to undergo chemo!"

Chapter 15
My Treatment Plan

My first meeting with Dr. Hoffman is scheduled for October 19th, so beforehand, I researched Google to familiarize myself with the practitioner's background and skill level. Pleased with what I find, I feel Dr. Denton has made a solid referral and that I'll be in good hands with Dr. Hoffman. So, when we meet, after exchanging greetings, I tell her she comes highly recommended by Dr. Denton. I also let her know I've had a chance to review her credentials and find them impressive. She thanks me and says, "Why don't we start by having you tell me what you know about your medical condition?"

"As you may know, I've been diagnosed with prostate cancer. Of the treatment options I was presented with, I elected to have a robotic prostatectomy. Following my surgery, my PSA level was 0.61, but after it began to rise, it was suspected that my prostate cancer had spread. Subsequently, I had a nuclear whole-body scan, revealing that the cancer had not spread to my bones. However, shortly after, I had a PSMA PET Scan, which unfortunately revealed cancer had spread to four areas of my body. Is that about right?"

"That's correct, Mr. Simmons, and it has also been confirmed that cancer has been found in a fifth area, an obturator node in your pelvic region."

Then, just as my heart sinks, she says,

"But your cancer is treatable. Your treatment plan will be changing, however."

"Does this mean I'll need to undergo chemotherapy?"

"No, not at this juncture, and we don't currently anticipate having to use radiation, either. So instead, your treatment will involve a pill called Abiraterone, which we'll use in conjunction with Prednisone, a steroid."

"So, I've gotten into the clinical trial?"

"Yes! You have."

"I'm having difficulty pronouncing it, but what is Abi..? and what does it do?"

"The generic name for Abiraterone is Zytiga (zy-tee-ga), so let's call it that to make it easier for you to say. Zytiga is a pill designed to lower your testosterone."

"So, by lowering my testosterone, we're basically "starving the cancer cells," if I understand what Dr. Denton told me."

"That's a good way of putting it."

"Why will I need to take a steroid?"

"The effect of Zytiga reducing your testosterone level could lead to tiredness, so we "counterbalance" that with a steroid."

"What are the side effects of Zytiga?"

"Well, one is hot flashes."

"I'm familiar with the side effect of hot flashes because my wife's uncle had to take shots for his prostate cancer, and it caused him to have hot flashes."

"They're called Lupron injections. I want to see how well you do with Zytiga first, so you may or may not have to have Lupron injections, but we'll see."

"That's right; it's called Lupron. Hopefully, I won't have hot flashes from the Zytiga and won't need the shots later, either."

"I want to get you started on your medication immediately, so I'll write up a prescription for you, and after I leave, I'll ask one of our pharmacists to sit with you to review your medications. Do you have any other questions?"

"Yes. How long will I have to be on Zytiga?"

"Probably, for the rest of your life."

Then, seeing the disappointment on my face, Dr. Hoffman adds, "Barring anything unforeseen, we expect you will live out your life expectancy. The reason why we must continue treating your cancer is to prevent it from coming back. Who knows? At some point, for example, say four or five years of your PSA level staying consistently at 0 or slightly above, you might ask me to come off the treatment. I've had patients request that before."

During our session, Dr. Hoffman also informs me that Emory Healthcare's genetics department offers DNA testing if I want to learn more about my genetic makeup. I tell her that her timing is perfect because I've been wondering if I inherited a gene for prostate cancer or if my case is a one-off. Subsequently, she tells me she'll have someone from the department contact me. (A week later, I met with two representatives of the Genetics department and ultimately had bloodwork done to determine if I had inherited a gene for prostate cancer.)

As we wrap up, Dr. Hoffman places my prescription order into a computer so I can begin my hormone treatment.

Then, when she says, "Mr. Simmons, it was a pleasure meeting you, I say, "The pleasure was all mine."

After about thirty minutes of waiting, a pharmacist hasn't come to see me, as Dr. Hoffman had said would happen, so I walk into the hallway and spot a nurse. I told her Dr. Hoffman told me a pharmacist was supposed to be coming to meet with me, but that was thirty minutes ago. The nurse apologizes and says, "Oh my goodness. Let me see what's going on. I'm so sorry for the inconvenience. What room are you in?" "Number 2," I say. She says, "Let me find out what's going on, and I'll come back to you with an update, Okay?" "Okay," I say.

About five minutes later, a pharmacist rushes into the exam room, frazzled and gasping for air. "I'm sorry you've had to wait so long, Mr. Simmons. Today has been an absolute zoo. I was in another building when I learned you were waiting to see a pharmacist. So I got over here as soon as possible," she says. "Not a problem," I say. After catching her breath, the pharmacist reviews my prescriptions with me and tells me how often I should take my medications. When she finishes, she hands me an information package containing more detail about what she's just covered.

When I get home, I Google Zytiga. I discover that not only has it been FDA-approved, but more than 3,000 men with metastatic prostate cancer, like mine, have participated in the clinical trial involving the drug. I'm pleased that a significant number of men have gone through the clinical trial already because I don't want to be a medical guinea pig. Nevertheless, it's strange, and I can't explain why I already strongly feel Zytiga will kill my remaining cancer.

I'm in a post-operation session with a nurse assistant six months following my prostate surgery. She types my answers into a computer when she asks me questions during the meeting. When she asks about my incontinence, I tell her I'm pleased with how well my physical therapy sessions (which she had prescribed two months earlier) are going. I also told her that I no longer wear incontinence underwear and returned to regular underwear and that my only problem was that when I laughed or sneezed, I would leak a small amount of urine. As we wrap up, the nurse assistant says, "So, Mr. Simmons, how are you doing with your erections?" The question wakes both my shoulder angels, so as they flap their wings, I suspect they're about to duke it out over how I respond to the nurse's inquiry. Anticipating the showdown, other angels form a ring and hover around the two. My right shoulder angel shadow-boxes to get ready to take on her polarizing counterpart. Following is a recap of their "bout."

Round 1

Left shoulder angel:

"Player, Player! You go, Butch. When a lady asks you how your erections are going, you have to ask if she's interested, Player! So, go ahead and ask her."

Right shoulder angel:

"Shut your wings, you ignoramus! (The angel crowd goes, Woo!). The woman is just doing her job by asking Butch that question following his prostate surgery."

Left shoulder angel:

"Yeah, doll. All I know is that the man wore a catheter for six months. So, I'm just helping out with what has to be pent-up demand."

Right shoulder angel:

Infuriated, the right shoulder angel throws a right-wing uppercut and knocks the left shoulder angel flat on his back. Walking back to her corner, the right shoulder angel says, "Take that for pent-up demand!"

Round 2

Left shoulder angel:

Wobbling back into the ring, he says, "Look, Butch, I've got you covered, brother. You don't need Viagra with me by your side, partner. You're a Mandingo warrior, so I'm telling you, if you don't go ahead and ask this woman if she's interested, I'm giving you another yeast infection!"

Right shoulder angel:

Coaxes the left shoulder angel into the middle of the ring, and the two start winging it out toe-to-toe. Feathers are flying everywhere, and the hovering angels are roaring their approval. Soon, the referee steps in to separate the two angels, and when he does, the left shoulder angel is bleeding in the groin area. He's been castrated by the right shoulder angel, so she wins by technical knockout (TKO), and Butch doesn't ask the nurse if she's interested.

THE END.

After fully recovering from my erection question, on November 3rd, I had bloodwork done at my nephrologist's office, Dr. Kumar, for my upcoming meeting with him on the 10th to see how my kidneys are doing. When he and I meet, my prior week's test results show my kidneys are functioning at 33%, over a fivefold improvement since my hospitalization. This development seems to surprise Dr. Kumar because as he's viewing my new numbers on a computer screen, his arms raised slightly, his back straightens, and his head jerks back as if saying, 'Wow!'

After that, he turns and looks at me and says, "Your numbers look great! When I first met you, I was certain you would have to be placed on dialysis." I reply, "You know what it is, right?" "No," he answers. "Many people have been praying for me," I tell him. "I believe it," he says. As I continue conversing with Dr. Kumar, he still seems confused about my kidneys' improvement. It's as if he's wondering if something out of the ordinary is happening with my body, something that can't be medically explained. Unfortunately, I don't have time to tell him about the bright light and the angel's wing because he has to run off to another appointment. But, I strongly think, like me, he's beginning to suspect something extraordinary is happening with my body. Considering everything I've been through, and my rapid health improvement, I'm starting to view myself as a "walking miracle."

Heading into the week before Thanksgiving, a courier delivers my Zytiga and Prednisone prescriptions. After opening their plastic containers, I was surprised by the size disparity between the pills. The brown Zytiga tablets look like "horse pills" and are so large one can barely fit, length-wise, into a compartment of my new pill dispenser. Conversely, the white Prednisone pills are so tiny that I'm afraid if I drop one, I probably won't be able to find it.

After placing my new medication in my pill dispenser, I pray that the Zytiga will work and "starve" my cancer so I'll be cancer-free soon. Per my prescription, I'll take two Zytiga tablets and one Prednisone pill daily. After being on my new medication for a few days, I'm managing to swallow the large Zytiga tablets without much complication, but I have gagged a few times due to their large size. While I didn't think I'd have any problem ingesting the tiny steroid pills, I struggled with their bitter aftertaste, which is far worse than an uncoated aspirin. And fortunately, I haven't experienced any of Zytiga's potential side effects, such as "hot flashes," frequent urination, muscle cramps, etc. One day I did feel a little "spaced out" after taking the medication, but I think it was brought on by taking a prescribed iron tablet on an empty stomach.

I can't quite put my finger on it, and it's hard to explain, but my insides feel like Zytiga is winning the "tug-of-war" with my prostate cancer. Perhaps that's just wishful thinking, but I'm feeling much stronger on the inside, and I don't believe it's related to my being on a steroid. I'm also experiencing what feels like an inner cleansing. I'm noticing I have more significant and stickier bowel movements. It's as if my entire system is being flushed of impurities. As I try to visualize what might be happening inside my body, it's as if a quiet war is raging, and Zytiga is winning and causing my prostate cancer and its contaminants to retreat.

On December 16th, I'm scheduled to meet with a nurse practitioner assisting Dr. Hoffman to discuss my PSA level and how Zytiga is doing against my prostate cancer. I'm cautiously optimistic and not nearly as nervous as I've been in my prior visits with Dr. Aminu and others when I'm about to receive an update on my status. However, I still can't shake the feeling that the drug is working and killing my cancer. When I arrived at the hospital, the receptionist told me I was in the wrong place and that my visit was in the building next door, where the sign reads Winship Cancer Institute of Emory University. So when I say, "The address in MyChart says I'm supposed to be here, now you're telling me I have to go right back to the building across from where I parked and just walked passed she bluntly replies, "Yes." Irritated, I head back down a hill to the building next door.

When I got inside, a receptionist told me to take the elevator to the first floor, where the Oncology department is located. 'That's strange,' I think. 'Why didn't I have blood work done to assess my PSA level first?' After I get upstairs to Oncology, my vitals are taken, and after a short wait, I meet with a nurse practitioner. After introducing herself, she looks at her computer screen, doesn't see my PSA lab results, and realizes a mistake has been made.

"Mr. Simmons, I'm so sorry. You were sent up here by mistake. I see what the problem is, however. Your bloodwork request was made at the last minute, and the reception area must not have seen the order. So, if you don't mind, please go back downstairs, have your bloodwork done, and come back here to Oncology."

"Yeah, at noon, there was no mention on MyChart that I was to have bloodwork done, then at 12:30, thirty minutes before I was supposed to be here, MyChart showed that I was scheduled for lab work. Immediately I knew something was wrong, so I made it here as fast as possible. When the receptionist told me to head upstairs, I figured my bloodwork would be done up here, so I didn't question where I was supposed to do the lab work. So, I'll head back downstairs."

"Great! I have another appointment scheduled, but I'm pushing it back since we've already inconvenienced you. I'll meet with you when you return upstairs and after your bloodwork has been processed, which should take about fifteen to twenty minutes."

"Okay, I'll see you in a bit," I say.

So when I hop onto the elevator to head back downstairs, I'm pretty pissed about the run around I've been given from the wrong building assignment to now this. So, as I'm fuming, my right shoulder angel whispers in my ear and says, 'Butch, you need to calm down. These people are stressed and overworked from the pandemic, and they're doing their best to help save your life, and here you are, upset. You need to give these people a break and take a chill pill. Life's too short to be worried about trivial stuff like this.' 'Yeah, you're right,' I inwardly reply to the angel. So by the time the elevator doors open, I've calmed down. Finally, I got my blood work done and returned to the first floor to meet with the nurse practitioner again. When she comes in, she says,

"Mr. Simmons, I'm so sorry about the mix-up today."

"No problem. The nurse got me in and out in just a few minutes. One of the nurses told me she thought it might take ten to fifteen minutes for my results to return. I had just finished checking MyChart before you came in, and I'm disappointed that the results aren't back after twenty minutes. I'm anxious to know if Zytiga is killing my prostate cancer cells."

"I understand, Mr. Simmons. It's not unusual for cancer patients to want to know their PSA results every month or immediately. We've learned, however, that PSA testing every three months provides better information on how Zytiga treatment is performing. So for the foreseeable future, we'll check your PSA level quarterly versus monthly. Today's lab work, however, is to assess your liver's response to the Zytiga treatment."

"Oh, I had completely forgotten that a potential side effect of Zytiga is possible liver damage. So how is my liver doing?"

"Your liver function looks fantastic, and there are no apparent adverse effects from the Zytiga. However, you will need monthly blood tests to monitor your liver. Hmm, I'm surprised you're not on Orgovyx. Did Dr. Hoffman mention it when you and she talked?"

"I don't recall. Is Orgovyx a pill used instead of a shot? If it is, I received mail from my insurance provider the other day saying the claim was denied."

"Oh, yes. I see that here now. What about Lupron? Did she mention that?"

"Yes, she did mention it. I understand I should only be on oral medication, though."

"I'm pretty sure you're supposed to be on Lupron too. It's an additional means to help lower your testosterone level. Give me a minute, and let me go and check with Dr. Hoffman."

So the nurse practitioner leaves and is gone for about five minutes. When she returns, she says, "Yes, Dr. Hoffman would like you to start Lupron treatment today. After we finish here, I'll have a nurse take you for your injection."

Although this latest development catches me off guard, inwardly, I think, 'Anything that will help eliminate this cancer inside my body, then I'm all for it.' When the nurse practitioner and I finish, she hands me off to another nurse who escorts me to the Lupron injection waiting area. After a short wait, a third nurse comes to get me and takes me into a large room about half the size of the hospital's lobby. About thirty to forty people, including nurses, are milling around or standing and talking. The aura of the place is bizarre; it feels like I just stepped into a sci-fi movie, with people just meandering around waiting to be cloned or something. I've never seen anything like this, so I think, 'What in the world! Are all these people here for Lupron shots? On second thought, I don't think I want one!'

The nurse takes me to a curtained area on my right and asks if I've ever had a Lupron injection. "No, I've never had one before. All I know about them is that one side effect is hot flashes, which I hope I won't have after I receive the injection," I tell her. Lupron injections aren't so bad," she says. "I was involved in an accident when I was young and had to take them for years. I would take them in my stomach. Where would you like to take yours?" 'Nowhere,' I'm thinking. But instead, I say, "What are my options?" She says, "You can take it in your stomach, the meaty part of the back of your arm, or your butt." My bravado kicks in, and I think, 'Well, if a little girl can take a Lupron injection in her stomach, so can I.' So, I boldly proclaim, "I'll have mine in my stomach. Now, what do I need to do next?" "Pull up your shirt for me and keep it up with your left hand. I want you to take your right hand and squeeze a fatty part of your stomach for me," she instructs me. So as I'm doing what the nurse says, she's priming her needle, which looks about two and a half inches long, and fluid squirts in the air as she does.

Looking at the long needle, I'm having second thoughts about a stomach shot. Maybe I should take the injection in the meaty part of the back of my arm or butt but not in my stomach. But since the nurse said she took the shots when she was a little girl, if I tell her I've changed my mind, she'll think I'm a wuss. So, I've got to gut this one out, pun intended. Next, the nurse inserts the long needle into my stomach, and I think, 'She must have been one tough little girl because this shit is hurting like hell!' After the nurse removes the needle, I say, "Phew!" Following the stomach injection, I vowed that the next time I take a Lupron shot, it would be in my arm or my butt, but not my stomach! Afterward, my abdomen was sore for two days.

Because of the scheduling mishap today, my appointment ran thirty minutes longer than expected. So when I leave the hospital, I get stuck in Atlanta's Friday rush hour traffic. Flustered when I get home, I notice an email in Outlook stating I have a message in MyChart. After I access the patient portal, there's a message from the nurse practitioner. I think, 'She's writing to apologize for the disruptions I experienced today.' So, when I opened the message, the nurse practitioner reported my PSA results came back after I left, and my level had dropped to 0.13! "Oh My God," I shout out. "It's working! The Zytiga is starving my cancer!" Also, a few hours later, my DNA test returned, and the results were negative regarding whether I inherited a gene for prostate cancer, so it turns out my cancer is an anomaly. I'm immensely relieved to learn I'm not a carrier of the gene because, as I understand, if I were, my sons would be susceptible to prostate cancer and my daughter to breast cancer. After both bits of good news, I start crying, and it takes me about fifteen minutes to compose myself. When I do, I call Bay with the good news, and she says, "God is so good," and I reply, "Yes, He is." After we get off the phone, I text Bay and the kids, recapping my day. Everyone is thrilled with my latest news.

Chapter 16
The Price I've Paid

I have paid a tremendous price physically, psychologically, and emotionally for allowing my "manhood" to stand in the way of annual rectal exams. In one (1) year and five (5) months, I've had sixty-eight (68) hospital and doctor's office-related events, some of which I list below. Financially, and as of this writing, my hospital bills have totaled **$255,363.96** and will continue to grow due to lab work, prescriptions, follow-up visits, etc. Fortunately, insurance has covered ninety-seven (97%) of the expense. Still, I've had to pay 3% of the amount, which is a shame because my entire prostate cancer scenario could have possibly been avoided altogether were it not for my healthcare negligence!

Description	Qty	Cost
Hospital Charges	1	$86,397.14
Robotic Prostatectomy	1	$68,295.93
Cystoscopy	3	$28,712.84
Pet Scan DSMA	1	$19,154.00
ER Physician Charges	1	$21,457.16
Emergency Room	1	$10,475.92
Nephrostomy Tubes	2	$8,191.81
Labwork,X-Rays,Zytiga	2	$4,941.16
MRI	2	$4,306.00
NM Whole Body Scan	2	$3,432.00
Total		$255,363.96

My medical expenses as of this writing

Some of My Prostate Cancer Events

- My kidney function was 6% GFR when I was admitted to the hospital. The emergency room doctor told me that if I had waited much longer, it was likely I might have had to have been placed on dialysis.

- 3 Cystoscopies followed by bilateral stent placements to help me urinate

- Pre-operation diagnosis - bilateral hydronephrosis, acute renal failure

- Renal bladder ultrasound

- Creatinine level reached 8.25 mg/dl. Note: A healthy range is 0.70 mg/dl - 1.30 mg/dl. In non-medical terms, my creatinine level was through the roof!

- Prostate-Specific Antigen (PSA) reached 46.59 ng/ml. This score is nine (9) times higher than the average for a Black man my age, per the National Library of Medicine)! Note: 3 months after my prostate surgery, my urologist wanted to see a level of less than 0.00 ng/ml.

- Bilateral nephrostomy tubes to provide drainage from my kidneys to my bladder

- 16-inch French Foley catheter placement after emergency room visit

- I failed four (4) urinary void trials to see if I could urinate on my own without the aid of a catheter

- Prostate biopsy and CT rectal exam. Twelve (12) tissue samples were taken from my prostate during the biopsy.

- 3D MRI to identify the cause of my urine blockage

- 2 Nuclear Medicine Whole Body Bone Scans to see if cancer had invaded my bones

- 25-pound weight loss over one year

- Robotic prostatectomy to remove cancerous prostate

- 40% of prostate had cancer

- Averaged two hours of sleep over four months

- I had to begin wearing urinary "diapers" due to incontinence following prostate surgery

- Wore a catheter for six months

Chapter 17
What's Next?

I don't know what comes next in my prostate cancer journey, but I'm encouraged that my PSA level is continuing to drop, 0.01 ng/ml on April 11, 2023, and that the "silent killer" inside me appears to be retreating. When I asked the bright light to look inside my heart and weigh the good things I've done versus the bad, it must have heard me and sent the right wing of an angel, perhaps my right shoulder one or my Mom; I don't know which, to watch over me. I know I'm a different person now than I was in November of 2021. I've learned to appreciate things more, such as my family, health, and life. Things that used to bother me don't worry me as much, and I have an inner peace I've never known before. I've also gained a far greater appreciation for people with cancer and pray for those who must undergo radiation treatment, or chemotherapy, wear a catheter, or self-catheterize daily. And my previous mindset that having a rectal exam would make me less of a man has been shattered to the core, and I've been awakened by the importance of seeing a doctor regularly. My ignorance and arrogance regarding rectal exams nearly cost me my life, and I've paid a severe price for my negligence.

The saddest part about my battle with prostate cancer is that it probably could have been avoided altogether. Had I known all I had to do was have bloodwork (i.e., a PSA test) to see how my prostate was doing, I would have done so without hesitating. Maybe my suffering was intended for me to share my experience so that other men might see the "light" about getting checked regularly for prostate cancer. I certainly have. So, I pray that my plight will motivate others to act, for if they do nothing, they could end up like me or worse.

Ironically, as I was finishing up this book, I received a call and a text from an old Auburn basketball teammate, Bernard Montgomery, who was trying to reach me to congratulate me on recently being appointed to the Board of Directors of the James Owens Foundation. During our conversation, I shared with Bernard that I have prostate cancer and am writing a book about my journey. He listened as I took him through some of the events I had experienced, and when I finished, he said, "Flea, my Auburn basketball nickname; I never told you this, but I've experienced prostate cancer too. Unfortunately, I had robotic surgery in 2005, when it was in its infancy. But, if it helps you, I'm still here, and that was 17 years ago. So, Get your book out!"

Bernard's words were most comforting because they gave me hope that I might have the same post-prostate surgery longevity as him. Eerily, when I picked up K.J. from work that same day because his car was in the shop for maintenance, I told him about my conversation with Bernard, and he said, "Dad, you've got to get that book out!" I've now received at least eight recommendations to share my prostate cancer experience with others. So, I'm convinced I should do so.

Hopefully, my prostate cancer journey will be helpful to others, and should they be impacted by the disease, I hope they, too, receive a bright light and the right wing of an angel to comfort them and give them hope in their time of need.

My Hope

If someone you know or love is hesitant about rectal exams, please encourage them to at least have bloodwork done to assess their PSA level. It could save their lives, and they could avoid potentially ending up like me.

References

- Memorial Sloan Kettering Cancer Center (MSK) – "3 Things Black Men Should Know about Prostate Cancer" (https://www.mskcc.org/news/things-black-men-should-know-about-prostate)

- Wikipedia
  - Rudy (film) - https://en.wikipedia.org/wiki/Rudy (film)
  - Creative Commons image of a Nephrostomy Tube Needleness Connector

- American Cancer Society – "Key Statistics for Prostate Cancer." (https://www.cancer.org/cancer/prostate-cancer/about/key-statistics.html#:~:text=Risk%20of%20prostate%20cance r,rare%20in%20men%20under%2040.)

- PLOS ONE - "Are You Your Friends' Friend? Poor Perception of Friendship Ties Limits the Ability to Promote Behavioral Change." (https://journals.plos.org/plosone/article?id=10.1371/journal.pone.0151588.)

Source	Reciprocal	Non-Reciprocal
Friends and Family dataset	45%	55%
Reality Mining dataset	34%	66%
Social Evolution dataset	35%	66%
Strongest Ties dataset	49%	51%
Personality Survey	53%	47%
MIT	53%	47%
Average	45%	55%

Average of six studies mentioned in the PLOS ONE article

Author Biography

Eric Simmons is the CEO of ESE, Inc., a website development firm specializing in creating sites for small businesses, high school/college athletes, authors, poets, and others who seek to project their "Personal Brand" on the Internet. A former college athlete, he enjoys sports and public speaking. He self-publishes under his full name, Eric Otis Simmons, and his written works are branded under the name ESETOMES (pronounced ESE-TOMES) to represent a "volume of books."

Eric has written and self-published four books that have appeared on Amazon's "Best Sellers" list 181 times since January 2019. His Memoir, "Not Far From The Tree," chronicles his life and underscores how his single mother's teachings propelled him to excel academically, athletically, and in Corporate America. "#HTSP - How to Self-Publish" is based on the steps he undertook to write, market, and distribute his Memoir. "Getting Your Book Into Libraries" evolved from his well-received article, "How To Get Your Book Into Libraries," which became the top Google search result, out of over 2 billion, on the subject of "getting your book into libraries." Over 200 Libraries have purchased Simmons' self-published books. "Self Publisher's Toolkit" is a two-in-one resource that shows the reader how to self-publish a book and market it to Libraries, a viable $30+ billion segment often overlooked by self publishers.

To learn more about Eric and his books, visit https://www.eseinc1.com/esetomes-books.

Social Media

- Facebook: www.facebook.com/esimmonsauthor

- Twitter: @esimmonsauthor